Baillière's
# CLINICAL
# OBSTETRICS
# AND
# GYNAECOLOGY
INTERNATIONAL PRACTICE AND RESEARCH

Baillière's

# CLINICAL OBSTETRICS AND GYNAECOLOGY

INTERNATIONAL PRACTICE AND RESEARCH

Volume 2/Number 3
September 1988

# Anti-hormones in Clinical Gynaecology

D. HEALY BMed Sci, MB BS, PhD, FRACOG
*Guest Editor*

Baillière Tindall
London Philadelphia Sydney Tokyo Toronto

Baillière Tindall    24–28 Oval Road,
W.B. Saunders        London NW1 7DX

The Curtis Center, Independence Square West,
Philadelphia, PA 19106–3399, USA

1 Goldthorne Avenue
Toronto, Ontario M8Z 5T9, Canada

Harcourt Brace Jovanovich Group (Australia) Pty Ltd,
32–52 Smidmore Street, Marrickville, NSW 2204, Australia

Exclusive Agent in Japan:
Maruzen Co. Ltd. (Journals Division)
3–10 Nihonbashi 2-chome, Chuo-ku, Tokyo 103, Japan

ISSN 0950–3552

ISBN 0–7020–1302–1 (single copy)

*Baillière's Clinical Obstetrics and Gynaecology* is published four times each year by Baillière Tindall. Annual subscription prices are:

| TERRITORY | ANNUAL SUBSCRIPTION | SINGLE ISSUE |
| --- | --- | --- |
| 1. UK & Republic of Ireland | £35.00 post free | £15.00 post free |
| 2. USA & Canada | US$68.00 post free | US$25.00 post free |
| 3. All other countries | £45.00 post free | £18.50 post free |

The editor of this publication is Seán Duggan, Baillière Tindall, 24–28 Oval Road, London NW1 7DX.

*Baillière's Clinical Obstetrics and Gynaecology* was published from 1983 to 1986 as *Clinics in Obstetrics and Gynaecology*.

Typeset by Phoenix Photosetting, Chatham.
Printed and bound in Great Britain by Mackays of Chatham PLC, Chatham, Kent.

# Contributors to this issue

**MARC BYGDEMAN** MD, PhD, Professor, Department of Obstetrics and Gynaecology, Karolinska Hospital, S-104 01 Stockholm, Sweden.

**IAIN T. CAMERON** BSc, MD, MRCOG, MRACOG, Senior Registrar, Royal Womens Hospital, 132 Grattan Street, Carlton, Victoria 3053, Australia.

**J. R. T. COUTTS** BSc, PhD, Reader in Reproductive Endocrinology, University Department of Obstetrics and Gynaecology, Glasgow Royal Infirmary, 10 Alexandra Parade, Glasgow G31 2ER, UK.

**CATHERINE DUBOIS** MD, Roussel-UCLAF, 35 bd des Invalides, 75007 Paris, France.

**R. FLEMING** BSc, PhD, Biochemist, University Department of Obstetrics and Gynaecology, Glasgow Royal Infirmary, 10 Alexandra Parade, Glasgow G31 2ER, UK.

**S. FRANKS** MD, FRCP, Senior Lecturer in Reproductive Endocrinology, Department of Obstetrics and Gynaecology, St Mary's Hospital Medical School, London W2 1PG, UK.

**HAMISH M. FRASER** PhD, DSc, Senior Scientist, MRC Reproductive Biology Unit, Centre for Reproductive Biology, 37 Chalmers Street, Edinburgh EH3 9EW, UK.

**B. J. A. FURR** BSc, PhD, Bioscience I, ICI Pharmaceuticals, Alderley Park, Macclesfield, Cheshire SK10 1LT, UK.

**DAVID L. HEALY** BMed Sci, MB BS, PhD, FRACOG, Honorary Senior Lecturer, Department of Obstetrics and Gynaecology, Monash University, Monash Medical Centre, 246 Clayton Road, Clayton, Victoria 3168, Australia.

**GARY D. HODGEN** PhD, The Jones Institute for Reproductive Medicine, Eastern Virginia Medical School, 855 West Brambleton Avenue, Suite B, Norfolk, Virginia 23510, USA.

**D. LYNN LORIAUX** MD, PhD, Developmental Endocrinology Branch, National Institute of Child Health and Human Development, National Institute of Health, Bethesda, Maryland, USA.

**K. MARK McKENNA** MB BS, MRACOG, Lecturer, Department of Obstetrics and Gynaecology, University of Melbourne, Royal Womens Hospital, Grattan Street, Carlton, Melbourne, Australia.

**LYNNETTE K. NIEMAN** MD, Developmental Endocrinology Branch, National Institute of Child Health and Human Development, National Institute of Health, Bethesda, Maryland, USA.

**R. J. PEPPERELL** MDBS, MGO, FRACP, FRCOG, FRACOG, Professor, Department of Obstetrics and Gynaecology, University of Melbourne, Royal Womens Hospital, Grattan Street, Carlton, Melbourne, Australia.

**M. J. REED** BSc, MSc, PhD, MRCPath, Senior Lecturer, Chemical Pathology, Department of Chemical Pathology, St Mary's Hospital Medical School, London W2 1PG, UK.

**ROBERT W. SHAW** MD, MRCOG, FRCS, Head, Academic Department of Obstetrics and Gynaecology, Royal Free Hospital School of Medicine, Pond Street, London NW3 2QG, UK.

**KENNETH A. STEINGOLD** MD, Medical College of Virginia, Department of Obstetrics and Gynaecology, Box 34, MCV Station, Richmond, Virginia 23298, USA.

**ANDRE ULMANN** MD, PhD, Roussel-UCLAF, 35 bd des Invalides, 75007 Paris, France.

**PAUL F. A. VAN LOOK** MD, PhD, Special Programme of Research, Development and Research Training in Human Reproduction, World Health Organization, 1211 Geneva 27, Switzerland.

**CHRISTINE P. WEST,** MBChB, MRCOG, Consultant Obstetrician and Gynaecologist and Honorary Senior Lecturer, Edinburgh Royal Infirmary and Centre for Reproductive Biology, 37 Chalmers Street, Edinburgh EH3 9EW, UK.

**E. CARL WOOD** CBE, MB BS, FRCS, FAGO, Chairman, Monash University, Department of Obstetrics and Gynaecology, Monash Medical Centre, 246 Clayton Road, Clayton 3168, Melbourne, Australia.

# Table of contents

**RECENT ISSUES**

March 1988
**Antenatal and Perinatal Causes of Handicap**
NAREN PATEL

June 1988
**Gynaecology in the Elderly**
STUART L. STANTON

**FORTHCOMING ISSUES**

December 1988
**Operative Treatment of Cervical Cancer**
E. BURGHARDT & J. M. MONAGHAN

March 1989
**Operative Treatment of Ovarian Cancer**
E. BURGHARDT & J. M. MONAGHAN

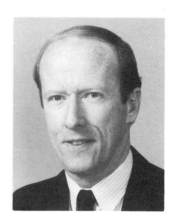

# Foreword

Modern gynaecology and obstetrics demands a blend of surgical, medical and psychological skills probably not matched in any other area of medicine. Furthermore, our specialty has been central in recent discussions concerning many of the ethical dilemmas of modern medicine. In this setting, selection of a series of authors to review recent advances in the application of anti-hormones to clinical gynaecological practice was an exciting challenge. The invited contributors have more than done justice to their briefs. The development and use of compounds that bind to specific hormone receptors but do not activate the subsequent intracellular events, so blocking the action of hormones and acting as anti-hormones, has significant impact for gynaecological practice.

In the first chapter, Wood discusses the societal implications of anti-hormone medicines in clinical gynaecology. This emphasis on the ethical and social aspects of these therapies sets the stage for the chapter by McKenna and Pepperell upon the use of anti-oestrogens in reproductive medicine. Furr then summarizes the current status of the use of anti-oestrogens in breast and gynaecological malignancies while Reed and Franks thoroughly review the place of anti-androgens in gynaecological practice.

The recent development of a series of compounds which bind to the progesterone receptor and antagonise progesterone action has major implications for gynaecological and obstetric practice. Cameron and Healy review the background and clinical physiology of these substances while Nieman and Loriaux discuss the use of anti-progesterones for the induction of menstruation in both animal models and human beings. It has been estimated that up to 100 000 women per year may die from surgical sepsis following termination of pregnancy in the third world. Accordingly, the development of non-surgical methods of safe termination of pregnancy may prevent such deaths and Bygdeman and Van Look review the current state of the art in using anti-progesterones for the interruption of established first trimester pregnancy. In addition to these uses, anti-progesterones may have wider applications in gynaecological and obstetric practice: Ulmann and Dubois discuss the potential roles of those in obstetrics, ectopic pregnancy and those gynaecological malignancies in which cancer growth appears associated with progesterone receptors and progesterone action.

The isolation of the hypothalamic hormone luteinizing hormone releasing hormone (LHRH) and the subsequent demonstration that continuous infusion of this hormone reduced, or down-regulated, pituitary follicle stimulating hormone (FSH) and luteinizing hormone (LH) secretion, rather than stimulated FSH and LH release, were seminal studies in reproductive medicine. They spawned extensive development of a range of LHRH agonist and antagonist compounds. The LHRH agonists have been extensively studied and Fraser has been a pioneer in elucidation of their clinical physiology and delivery systems. Shaw comprehensively reviews the current place of LHRH agonists in the management of endometriosis where suppression of pituitary followed by suppression of ovarian function was a new concept in the management of this common gynaecological disease.

Another common gynaecological problem, polycystic ovary syndrome, is still not completely understood although Fleming and Coutts have been instrumental in using LHRH agonists to suppress the disordered FSH and LH secretion in this disease and to thereby provide a new modality of treatment for this condition. Perhaps apart from skin tumours in Australian women, uterine leiomyomata (fibroids) represent the most common tumour in the human female. Despite this, our understanding of the pathogenesis of these neoplasms is poor and the treatment of uterine leiomyomata has traditionally been surgical. With the advent of modern ultrasonography, which allows the diagnosis of fibroids to be made more positively by the exclusion of ovarian masses, have come reports indicating that LHRH agonists will shrink uterine fibroids. The avoidance of surgery by the alternative use of implant injections of LHRH agonists is appealing to most patients and West has been instrumental in the pursuit of this aim. Finally, future directions in the research and clinical applications of anti-hormones to gynaecology and obstetrics are reviewed by Steingold and Hodgen in a scholarly contribution.

Additional gynaecological and obstetric uses for anti-hormones will continue to flow from the application of this concept to our discipline. The development of oxytocin receptor antagonists is one such example which is now being used as an oxytocin inhibitor for suppressing pre-term labour. Similar use of prostaglandin receptor antagonists may shortly follow. Furthermore, the recognition that the biological action of the glycoprotein hormones, such as FSH, depend not only on the polypeptide backbone of the hormone but also on the attached carbohydrate moieties indicates that the development of deglycosylated FSH isoforms with antagonistic activity may soon be feasible on a large scale. The extremely rapid progress in these areas will continue to pose new ethical dilemmas for gynaecologists and obstetricians and their patients.

I am indeed grateful to all the contributors to this volume for their chapters. I am also indebted to the considerable assistance provided by Sister Susan Bishop and for the secretarial excellence of Tricia Martin and Penny Ashley.

DAVID L. HEALY

# 1

# Anti-hormones in obstetrics and gynaecology: ethical and social issues

E. CARL WOOD

Gynaecology arose as a subspecialty of general surgery. Since then medical gynaecology has become increasingly important and relevant to the practice of the specialty. Drug therapy has reduced the need for certain surgical procedures such as uterine curettage and hysterectomy. The medicalization of gynaecology will increase with the development of anti-hormones. This evolution in reproductive medicine has been facilitated by the development of compounds which prevent the action of hormones on receptor sites so that physiological or pathophysiological systems can be modified. Because this development has been relatively recent, one can predict advances not yet addressed in the current volume. As the hormonal factors influencing a wider variety of diseases are better understood, so will the application of anti-hormones widen. Also it is not unreasonable to predict that hormone receptor sites may be blocked selectively in organs by binding anti-hormones to chemicals targeting to specific organ sites.

Anti-progesterones currently have the most important clinical application of anti-hormones. They can be used to induce menstruation or abortion. Therapeutic abortion is a community issue, particularly when it is controlled by the medical profession. When illegal, it is often carried out in unsatisfactory circumstances leading to ill health or even death. A change from surgical termination to medical termination has social implications. At the present time medical abortion is under medical control. If and when medical termination is judged simple and safe it will be more difficult to retain control of the procedure by the medical profession. While pharmaceutical companies produce anti-progesterones, governments can control the distribution of drugs, either by the medical profession or the pharmaceutical industry. However, when chemical manufacture is simplified it is likely that such drugs will flood local and overseas markets and be out of the control of government agencies. This may be to the advantage of poorer people in developed countries who may not be able to afford medical care, and would be much more advantageous to people in less developed countries who may have no access to medical care or alternatively have access to a poor standard of medical care. Once medical abortion is judged to be the appropriate equivalent of surgical abortion, it would profit hundreds of thousands of women to have ready access to medical abortion. Deaths from induced abortion, and the costs and sequelae of unskilled abortion would be reduced, and family planning programmes in countries where population growth is a serious economic disadvantage would be more effective.

Medical termination of pregnancy may also affect the clinical pattern of therapeutic abortion. Abortion may be done earlier because of the exclusion of complex protocols and hospital procedures and the ready availability of a drug in a nearby pharmacy. There would be less anxiety for the woman seeking abortion, a process which often delays the patient if she has to arrange medical care. Earlier abortion is safer abortion, as haemorrhage, infection and uterine trauma are less likely.

Abortion may be more easily obtained on demand, because if the drug was readily available, government policies determining the reasons for allowing therapeutic abortion would be difficult to police. The only system of control would be by close supervision of the drug supply and outlets. This difficulty would please 'pro-abortion' groups, but not those seeking to limit the procedure. Minors may also have more ready access to abortion, because, like marijuana, abortion pills could be supplied at school, even if the prices reflect those of a black market source.

Menstrual induction is available surgically but has not become popular because of the need to undergo a surgical procedure when one is uncertain of the existence of pregnancy. The possibility of an unnecessary surgical procedure, and the associated risk of sepsis when done in countries where pelvic infection is common, makes its application limited. Drug-induced menstrual induction has the advantage of having less risk of infection and having less effect on everyday life. The concept of preventive drug therapy, whether pregnancy exists or not, is consonant with other drug therapies taken to reduce the risk of illness.

Menstrual induction does raise new ethical issues. Is the induction of menstruation in the uncertain knowledge of pregnancy comparable to therapeutic abortion? It cannot be a criminal offence in a country where abortion is illegal, as there can be no proof that abortion has taken place. On the other hand there is a clear ethical implication that a person may have been pregnant when utilizing the technique. Anxiety and guilt may be reduced because of the uncertainty of the occurrence of pregnancy and the early state of embryo development. Nevertheless there may be women who become infertile and who may fantasize with regret about pregnancies lost by previous menstrual induction. The moral status of the early embryo is relevant. Embryos lost by menstrual induction are microscopic in size, unable to feel, a mass of cells, prone to early death, and not protected by legal sanctions. The recommendation of the Warnock Committee in the United Kingdom to allow embryo experimentation on the human embryo up to 14 days may reflect a community view that the moral status of the human embryo is less before 14 days than after this time (DHSS, 1984). Thus menstrual induction may become the preferred method of pregnancy termination. It would have ethical advantage over therapeutic abortion in those countries believing there is a gradual increase in the moral status of the human life between conception and birth.

Women may view anti-hormones in different ways. The ability to control some body functions by medication rather than surgical procedures, which are under close medical control, would be an advantage. Self-control of pregnancy and menstrual function would be an advantage. Drugs are viewed suspiciously by some and the term anti-hormone has the implication that one is interfering with nature. Education is the best counter to this fear. Side-effects of anti-hormones may be a disadvantage. When these are short-term and readily explained, such as with anti-progesterones, their concerns should not hinder their use. The possibility of more subtle long-term effects when using luteinizing hormone releasing hormone (LHRH) agonists or antagonists has still to be considered. Osteoporosis secondary to chronic oestrogen suppression by establishing a temporary medical menopause using LHRH agonists is one concern. The testing of possible long-term effects of drugs before widespread clinical usage has improved.

The control of parturition by anti-hormones may prevent premature labour or facilitate the termination of labour. While the prevention of premature labour has not been achieved it is possible that anti-hormones placed strategically in the cascade of events that determine uterine contractions may be effective either singly or in association with other substances. As prematurity is acknowledged as a major cause of perinatal death and morbidity, the development of such compounds does not require ethical justification because of obvious humane and economic advantages. The important social and ethical issue is how best the world can recruit resources to help speed the development of such compounds.

The termination of pregnancy may be required for obstetric reasons, but in some countries is used for the social convenience of the patient or medical attendant. If anti-hormones are able to produce a more physiological induction of labour without harm to the fetus or mother, social reasons for the induction of labour may become more acceptable. Precise timing of birth would help the woman who has a family or works, and improve the organization of obstetric services and the standard of clinical care.

LHRH agonists and antagonists have extended the science of ovulation induction, whether for the anovulatory or the in vitro fertilization patient. The method of delivery for temporary suppression of pituitary–ovarian function by a nasal spray or snuff avoids the need for injections and reduces the number of visits to hospital. Long-term suppression of pituitary–ovarian function by one injection of a LHRH agonist implant is rapidly becoming a reality. The ability to block ovarian function by using LHRH agonists or antagonists will assist many. The reduction in size of fibromyomata using these drugs may reduce the need for myomectomy, increase the safety of myomectomy and avoid hysterectomy.

The cure and control of endometriosis by LHRH inhibition of ovarian function is a suitable alternative to danazol therapy; this drug is not tolerated by many women. Long-term control of endometriosis may be improved by reducing ovarian function but not to the low level required to cure the disease. Control of excessive menstrual loss may also be possible by using anti-hormones to reduce oestrogen output. Contraception may be improved by anti-hormones. The action of endogenous oestrogen and progesterone could be manipulated to provide an unfavourable environment for the occurrence of ovulation, gamete transport or embryo implantation.

This book groups those areas of reproductive medicine where anti-hormones may be important. It is in many ways a view of the future of gynaecology.

## REFERENCES

Department of Health and Social Security (1984) *Report of Committee of Enquiry into Human Fertilization and Embryology. Chairman: Dame Mary Warnock*, Cmnd No 9314. London: Her Majesty's Stationary Office.

# 2

# Anti-oestrogens: their clinical physiology and use in reproductive medicine

K. MARK McKENNA
R. J. PEPPERELL

In the 28 years since the first clinical trials of treatment with clomiphene citrate this agent has become established as the standard treatment for women with anovulatory disorders due to hypothalamic dysfunction who wish to become pregnant. In well chosen patients it can be expected that over 80% will ovulate and that at least half of these will achieve a pregnancy. Clomiphene is also used widely in ovulatory women during controlled hyperstimulation for in vitro fertilization (IVF) and associated procedures. Despite this widespread use there are still many unresolved questions concerning its mode of action and the clinical physiology.

## Definitions

Only those substances that exert their action (or were thought to exert their action) through binding to the oestrogen receptor will be considered. Clearly other substances may exert an anti-oestrogenic effect by interfering with the action of oestrogens in target tissues—the action of prolonged progesterone treatment on the endometrium is a commonly seen clinical example. Similarly luteinizing hormone releasing hormone (LHRH) analogues may exert some of their effects by down-regulation of oestrogen receptors.

Clomiphene is the commonest anti-oestrogen used in reproductive practice, although other similar substances are in clinical use, including tamoxifen. In general this discussion of anti-oestrogens will concern clomiphene except where otherwise indicated.

## Structure

The anti-oestrogens do not have a steroidal structure. A steroidal configuration is not necessary for oestrogenic action, as evidenced by the highly potent non-steroidal oestrogens, such as diethylstilbestrol. The anti-oestrogens are triphenylethylene derivatives consisting of three phenyl groups and another group (a chloride moiety in clomiphene) attached to the ethyl double carbon, double bond core. The alkylether side chain on the phenyl groups may contribute to anti-oestrogen, anti-tumour activity (Murphy and Sutherland, 1983).

Some of these structures, such as chlorotrianisene, have a weak oestrogenic action.

## MODE OF ACTION

In general the anti-oestrogens can be thought of as competitors with oestradiol for their receptor and most actions in infertility treatment can be explained on this basis. In clinical practice it is satisfactory to have a concept of action of the anti-oestrogen at the hypothalamic–pituitary axis, resulting in an elevation of gonadotrophins enhancing follicular maturation. As might be expected the true situation is somewhat more complex.

### Effects at receptor level

It is clear that clomiphene interacts with the same receptor as oestradiol (Skidmore et al, 1972). Clarke et al (1974) showed that the anti-oestrogenic action was not due to simple competition for the receptor. They demonstrated that the anti-oestrogens tested, including clomiphene, were initially oestrogenic, stimulating rat uterine growth in the model used. Subsequently the action of the drugs was antagonistic because of a failure of replenishment of the receptor. The concept of drugs acting as agonists then antagonists on the reproductive pathways is now familiar.

Clomiphene citrate acts as an oestrogen rather than an anti-oestrogen at the level of the pituitary gonadotrophs, with an increased responsiveness in vitro to LHRH (Hsueh et al, 1978). Similarly the demonstration that calcium loss is retarded in oophorectomized monkeys given prolonged courses of clomiphene suggests an oestrogenic action (Abbasi and Hodgen, 1986). It may be that, as with the LHRH analogues, the dose, route and timing of administration may be as important as the drug itself.

To confuse matters further it is likely that specific anti-oestrogen receptors exist which are entirely different to the oestradiol receptor (Murphy and Sutherland, 1983). Five anti-oestrogens were tested for anti-tumour activity: their growth inhibitory actions were shown to be reversed by oestradiol when they had been given in low dose, but unaffected or only partly reversed at higher dosage. Tamoxifen has been shown to bind to a high-affinity saturable site which does not bind natural or synthetic oestrogens. It is likely that this 'anti-oestrogen' receptor binds to the side chains of the non-steroidal anti-oestrogens. This study demonstrated that zuclomiphene (previously designated the cis isomer) had a much higher affinity for the anti-oestrogen binding site than enclomiphene (trans isomer), which appeared to have a higher affinity for the oestrogen receptor. It also demonstrated that where the aromatic portion of the anti-oestrogens is held constant, modifications in the alkylether side chain affect the affinity for the oestrogen receptor. It is not clear whether the anti-oestrogen class of receptors has any role in the reproductive biology field.

### Effects on the hypothalamus and pituitary

Following the administration of clomiphene citrate there is a clear increase in luteinizing hormone (LH) and a rise in follicle-stimulating hormone (FSH) (Kerin et al, 1985), although the magnitude and existence of the FSH rise are controversial (Littman and Hodgen, 1985). The evidence from Yen's group (Hsueh et al, 1978) that clomiphene caused a sensitization of pituitary gonadotrophs to LHRH in vitro seemed to indicate that the anti-oestrogens were acting largely at the pituitary level. However it is known that clomiphene may cause hot flushes in the premenopausal woman and that it may antagonize the effects of oestrogen used to alleviate flushes in the menopause (Kauppila et al, 1981).

Kerin et al (1985) investigated women treated with clomiphene and demonstrated an increase in the pulse frequency of LH and FSH without an alteration in the pulse magnitude of these hormones. Pituitary sensitivity to LHRH as tested by LHRH challenge did not alter. This study, unlike many earlier ones, was placebo-controlled. It appears that the action of the anti-oestrogens in enhancing fertility is to increase the LHRH pulse frequency by an action at the hypothalamus (assuming that a change in pulsatility will be due to a hypothalamic mechanism). These findings have been confirmed by Judd et al (1987). Ayers et al (1987) have shown that in women over 35 years of age the increase in pulse frequency is not seen.

The assumption that the hypothalamus is the seat of clomiphene action because of this demonstrated effect on LH pulsatility may not be entirely correct. The presumption that pulsatility is a hypothalamic attribute has been questioned by recent work from the La Jolla group (Gambacciani et al, 1987) illustrating an intrinsic high-frequency, low-amplitude LH pulsatility in the isolated pituitary in vitro.

Using the cycling cynomolgus monkey as a model, Littman and Hodgen (1985) were unable to show an increase in FSH in response to clomiphene, although there was a significant rise in LH. It is possible that a rise in FSH was not seen because ovulatory animals were used and because daily hormone assays were used rather than the more frequent assays of Kerin's study which were able to look at individual pulses of gonadotrophins. These workers also showed that the mid-cycle LH surge was delayed in the clomiphene-treated group despite a more rapid oestradiol ($E_2$) rise to a higher level in this group. This suggests that clomiphene inhibits the positive feedback of oestradiol on LH towards mid-cycle as well as the negative feedback earlier in the cycle. In some cycles transient high LH levels were associated with a subsequent fall in $E_2$, which suggests that there may have been follicle atresia. While some believe that high levels of LH are associated with poor follicular development (Stanger and Yovich, 1985) others have reported no correlation between LH levels and outcome in a series of 845 patients in an established IVF programme (Thomas et al, 1987). The final answer on this is awaited with interest; however, the role of LH as a follicular poison is not established!

## Effects on the ovary

Marut and Hodgen (1982) found a fall in oestradiol with high-dose clomiphene despite an elevation in gonadotrophins in ovulatory rhesus monkeys. This suggests a direct ovarian effect in this model. In contrast, Kessel and Hsueh (1987) demonstrated a direct ovarian effect of clomiphene in vitro. Using a rat granulosa cell model the authors established that clomiphene augments FSH-mediated LH receptor formation, having previously shown a similar effect on FSH-stimulated aromatase activity. The action of clomiphene in augmenting FSH-mediated LH receptor production is not additive to that of oestradiol so it is likely the oestrogen receptor is the mediator of this oestrogen-like anti-oestrogen action.

Effects on the oocyte itself have also been suggested. Yoshimura et al (1985), using an isolated perfused rabbit ovary, found an increased incidence of germinal vesicle breakdown when clomiphene was perfused. This adverse effect could be opposed by the addition of human chorionic gonadotrophin (hCG) and oestradiol. Oestradiol also opposed an adverse effect on embryo development in this model (Yoshimura et al, 1987a). The same group (Yoshimura et al, 1986) demonstrated with the same model that fertilized ova from a clomiphene-perfused group were less likely to develop to the morula stage. In a further study (Yoshimura et al, 1987b) they reported that exposure to clomiphene reduced the number of offspring when the oocytes which had been ovulated in vitro were transferred; this effect could be abolished by the administration of oestradiol as above. Although interesting, the relevance of these data to the human is not at all certain. It should also be pointed out that gonadotrophins, in the absence of anti-oestrogens, have been shown to have similar effects on oocyte and embryo quality (Sato and Marrs, 1986; Vanderhyden et al, 1986).

## Effects on the endometrium

It is likely, but not at all certain, that there is no specific endometrial abnormality associated with the use of clomiphene, in the absence of an inadequate luteal phase. Lamb et al (1972) found no abnormality in luteal phase biopsies subjected to light microscopic examination. Baird's group (Thatcher et al, 1988) examined the endometrium of clomiphene-treated and control cycles and found no specific deleterious effect of the anti-oestrogen. They did note minor differences in mitotic rate and basal vacuolation of glandular epithelium. There was a correlation between less vacuolation and lower pregnanediol excretion in the clomiphene-treated patients. A lower mitotic index in the clomiphene-treated group suggests an inhibition of the mitogenic effect of oestradiol.

Fukuma et al (1983) found increased glycogen content, as well as increased glycogen synthetase and glycogen phosphorylase levels, in the endometrium of infertile women treated with clomiphene compared to a control cycle in the same woman. This was strongly correlated with mid-luteal levels of oestradiol and progesterone. They suggested that clomiphene improved the function of the corpus luteum and endometrium.

Birkenfeld et al (1986) reported on endometrial biopsies in the follicular phase after clomiphene treatment and demonstrated local or diffuse signs of early secretory change in 10 of 19 patients in the absence of elevated progesterone levels. This does suggest a direct effect but its significance as to pregnancy potential in a clomiphene-treated cycle is unclear.

The present authors have recently embarked on a cross-over study where primate embryos from clomiphene-stimulated animals are transferred to non-stimulated animals or the reverse procedure is carried out. We hope that this and similar studies may determine whether there is an adverse endometrial or oocyte/embryo factor associated with clomiphene use in the primate.

### Effects on cervical mucus

There is a clear effect of clomiphene on cervical mucus. It is important that studies considering this should be controlled as more than 20% of women may have a cervical score (Insler score) of less than 9, even following 4 days of treatment with 150 µg ethinyloestradiol per day (Insler et al, 1972; McBain and Pepperell, 1980). Lamb and Guderian (1966) reported poor mucus during treatment but also pointed out that the mucus usually improved before ovulation occurred. They emphasized that frequent examinations were necessary to observe this change and it is our experience that with daily examinations the mucus pattern is often seen to improve as long as there is adequate follicular development. O'Herlihy et al (1982) reported poorer cervical scores in clomiphene cycles than control cycles but again showed an improvement in cervical score as ovulation approached. Gysler et al (1982) reported that mucus was poor at post-coital testing in 15% of women ovulating in response to clomiphene. The use of low dose cis-clomiphene from days 2 to 27 of the cycle was suggested as a contraceptive measure by Pandya and Cohen (1972) because of the effect of this treatment on cervical mucus; it is interesting that a higher dose was not as effective.

## PHARMACOLOGY

Clomiphene citrate is supplied as a mixture of two isomers. The original designation of the cis and trans isomers was shown to be mistaken (that is, the cis isomer actually had a trans structure) and they have been renamed zuclomiphene and enclomiphene respectively. As discussed previously, these drugs have differing affinities for both oestrogen and anti-oestrogen receptors. Zuclomiphene appears to be the important isomer in ovulation induction; it seems that 10 mg zuclomiphene is equivalent clinically to 50 mg clomiphene citrate (Van Campenhout et al, 1973). Although Van Campenhout and co-workers suggest that the pregnancy rate may be higher with cis-clomiphene in a study on 37 patients, this is not supported in other studies (Charles et al, 1969; MacLeod et al, 1970; Connaughton et al, 1974).

There is an enterohepatic circulation of clomiphene metabolites; studies with radioactive tracer show that the drug is still present in faeces 6 weeks after administration. Using a radioreceptor assay Geier et al (1987) have shown that clomiphene or its metabolites is still present in the circulation on day 14 when given from days 5 to 9 of the cycle for ovulation induction. In some patients ligands were still present on day 22 but none were present 60 days after treatment.

### Side-effects and adverse effects

In a series of over 4000 anovulatory patients treated with clomiphene reported in 1968 by MacGregor et al, the commonest side-effects were ovarian enlargement (13.9%) followed by hot flushes (10.7%), pelvic or abdominal discomfort (7.4%), nausea (2.1%), breast discomfort (2.1%), visual symptoms (1.6%) and headache (1.1%). Side-effects occurring in less than 1% of patients include increased urination, depression, weight gain, allergic reactions and reversible hair loss.

While massive ovarian enlargement may occur rarely, the abdominal discomfort and breast symptoms are encouraging signs suggesting that ovulation is being achieved and, if explained as such, may be viewed positively by the patient. Vasomotor symptoms of hot flushes are also a good prognostic sign as regards ovulation (Lamb and Guderian, 1966). Visual symptoms seem to be reversible over weeks or days and may be due to intensification and prolongation of after-images (MacGregor et al, 1968). The occurrence of these visual symptoms is usually considered to contra-indicate further clomiphene treatment.

Although some early reports suggested high rates of spontaneous abortion in clomiphene-treated cycles, the abortion rate does not appear to be higher than in a similar infertile population. Similarly, some early case reports suggested an increased risk of neural tube defect; however, subsequent reports do not confirm an increase in any abnormality. The relevant studies concerning both miscarriage and malformations are listed by Kennedy and Adashi (1987). The combined reports of Kurachi et al (1983), Harlap (1976) and Gysler et al (1982) contain 1263 babies delivered after clomiphene treatment with no difference in anomalies compared to control groups. MacGregor et al (1968) report 1744 completed pregnancies with a 2% incidence of 'birth defects', but without a control group or clear definition of abnormality.

The similarity of the anti-oestrogens to the non-steroidal oestrogens has been noted earlier, as has the partly oestrogenic action of these compounds. It is therefore not surprising that Cunha et al (1987) demonstrated that tamoxifen and clomiphene had effects similar to diethylstilbestrol in genital tract tissue from aborted fetuses, grown in athymic mice treated with these drugs in a dose of 1–2 g/kg by pellet. The question of clinical importance is not whether the equivalent of over 1000 tablets given during a pregnancy is harmful, but whether subtle effects such as those that have followed diethyl-stilbestrol exposure in utero may occur when clomiphene is given before conception in normal dose. Studies of the long-term health and reproductive performance of the children of clomiphene-induced pregnancies are awaited with interest. There is currently no reason why clomiphene should not be used with the expectation that normal children will 'result; however, it should only be used in appropriate dosage, for appropriate indications and withheld if pregnancy cannot be excluded.

In the authors' own practice we have a small number of women with true ovarian resistance who appear to have re-entered a resistant high-gonadotrophin phase when clomiphene was given in an attempt to induce ovulation. We are unaware of any controlled studies in such patients but generally do not use clomiphene in these uncommon patients.

Multiple pregnancies occur in approximately 7% of patients (Asch and Greenblatt, 1976). As this rate consists of 6% twins and only 1% higher multiples this incidence is usually quite acceptable to physicians and patients.

## THE CLINICAL USE OF CLOMIPHENE

### Indications

It has been clear from the earliest reports of the use of clomiphene that it is most successful in inducing ovulation where there is adequate endogenous oestrogen production (MacGregor et al, 1968). This corresponds to the clinical situations of oligomenorrhoea or amenorrhoea where there is a progesterone withdrawal bleed. The patient may be obese, hirsute and have dysfunctional uterine bleeding. Generally, clomiphene is the treatment of choice in the polycystic ovarian syndrome where pregnancy is desired, though most cases will not have the classic Stein–Leventhal appearance. Hypo-oestrogenic women are less likely to respond to the anti-oestrogen treatment, although some do: 12 of 41 women who failed to bleed after medroxyprogesterone acetate ovulated in response to the first cycle of treatment with clomiphene in one study (Corenblum and Taylor, 1987). In clinical practice we use clomiphene before considering pulsatile GnRH or gonadotrophins, because less intensive management is necessary and the incidence of side-effects, particularly multiple pregnancy, is less.

In oligo-ovulation, where the cycles are 6 or more weeks in duration, there is a case for clomiphene treatment to allow more ovulatory cycles to occur in a defined time period and to prospectively define more accurately the actual time of ovulation.

While originally used with some success in the treatment of amenorrhoea–galactorrhoea cases (MacGregor et al, 1968), specific treatment with bromocriptine is preferred for the treatment of hyperprolactinaemic patients and has a much higher success rate for ovulation induction and pregnancy. Occasionally clomiphene may be needed to induce ovulation in hyperprolactinaemic patients who remain anovulatory on maximal doses of bromocriptine. Where the prolactin level has been suppressed to normal, the starting dose of clomiphene should be low; where the prolactin level is still elevated larger doses are required.

Although luteal phase defect has been described as a complication of clomiphene treatment (Garcia et al, 1977), it appears to be a useful treatment for this problem (Downs and Gibson, 1983; Huang, 1986).

The use of clomiphene in hyperstimulation regimens for IVF and associated procedures will be discussed briefly later.

### Standard treatment regimen

The patient is assessed before treatment to exclude thyroid disease, hyperprolactinaemia, hypergonadotrophic hypogonadism and pregnancy. As discussed later, there is a place for checking 17-hydroxyprogesterone (17OHP) or dehydroepiandrosterone sulphate (DHEAS) levels to exclude an adrenal defect, particularly if hirsutism is part of the clinical picture. The need to check the FSH level has been questioned (Grunert, 1984). However it should be considered important in women who fail to have a progesterone withdrawal bleed, who are over 35 years of age or who fail to respond to clomiphene. Due to the effects of unopposed oestrogen on the endometrium, sampling of the endometrium may be indicated, especially in the older woman with abnormal bleeding, because of the increased risk of endometrial atypia and carcinoma in this group of patients.

Although an assessment of the semen and a test for tubal patency are often deferred if there is no suggestion of an abnormality on history and physical examination, if pregnancy has not occurred after six clomiphene-induced ovulatory cycles these factors must be assessed.

Clomiphene is usually started in a dose of 50 mg/day for 5 days from day 5 of a natural cycle, or following a progestagen-induced withdrawal bleed. We use norethisterone or medroxyprogesterone acetate to initiate this bleed, and usually exclude pregnancy before administering the progestagen. This is not necessary in the patient in whom you are certain ovulation (including late ovulation) has not occurred. In patients with a clinical picture of classic polycystic ovarian syndrome we usually start treatment with clomiphene in a dose of 25 mg/day to avoid overstimulation (Dodge et al, 1986). Treatment is monitored using a single 24-h urinary collection for total urinary oestrogens and pregnanediol excretion in the mid-luteal phase. The use of this assay is discussed in the section on monitoring, below.

Commencing treatment on day 5 of the cycle has a rational basis following Hodgen's demonstration (Hodgen et al, 1985) that in the primate the dominant follicle is determined by day 5. Although this may not be the case in the anovulatory human, it is reasonable to delay treatment to this stage to reduce the risk of stimulating more than one dominant follicle. Despite this, it has been shown that where clomiphene is used as the sole agent for stimulation for IVF, a day 5 start results in higher oocyte numbers than a start on days 3, 4 or 7 (Marrs et al, 1984).

**Results of standard treatment with clomiphene citrate**

A series of large studies have shown that over 80% of patients will ovulate and that some 40–50% of patients treated will become pregnant (Garcia et al, 1977; Gysler et al, 1982; Chong et al, 1987). The discrepancy between ovulation and pregnancy rates has led to the suggestion that there is some factor associated with clomiphene treatment that decreases the chance of pregnancy in an ovulatory cycle. This factor has been suggested to be the effect on cervical mucus, the occurrence of unruptured luteinized follicles, the induction of a luteal phase defect, a toxic effect on the oocyte or embryo, or a toxic effect on the endometrium.

It is quite possible that the impression of a lower pregnancy rate is an error. Lamb et al (1972) demonstrated that the pregnancy rate per ovulatory cycle was similar to that in previously fertile women who have an intrauterine contraceptive device removed. They found no difference in the incidence of an unruptured luteinized follicle or of luteal phase defect in clomiphene or control cycles. Similar findings are outlined by Talbert (1983) and Hammond et al (1983). A recent review deals in more detail with this area (Kennedy and Adashi, 1987). A number of the early studies base the diagnosis of ovulation on temperature alone, which may be inaccurate. Many early studies include only three treatment cycles, as this was the recommended treatment at that time. While most pregnancies do occur in the first three treatment cycles (Rust et al, 1973; Gysler et al, 1982), in the study reported by Rust et al 35% of the total pregnancies occurred after the third cycle. A further confounding factor is that associated infertility problems are often discovered when further investigations are performed after clomiphene has failed to produce a pregnancy; if these cases are excluded high pregnancy rates are seen in ovulatory patients (Rust et al, 1974; Gysler et al, 1982).

More recently it has been suggested that the high pregnancy rate in frozen embryo replacement cycles may indicate an anti-pregnancy factor in the stimulated cycle (Testart et al, 1986). A review of 120 frozen embryo replacement cycles in our institution from January 1987 reveals a pregnancy rate of 24.1%. Of 131 cycles in which oocytes were frozen during this period 40 patients (30.5%) became pregnant in the index cycle. Although fewer embryos are transferred in the frozen embryo replacement group, the clear suggestion is that this subgroup of patients has a relatively high fertility. Patient selection is probably more important than clomiphene administration.

## What results can be expected in the individual patient?

An estimate of the probable success of clomiphene therapy in inducing ovulation and conception may be made before treatment starts. Important factors in this prognosis (assuming no other factors causing infertility are active) are the patient's weight, the underlying cause of her infertility and her basal oestrogen status.

Gysler et al (1982) reported an ovulation rate of 93% in patients with oligomenorrhoea and 62% in amenorrheoic patients with polycystic ovarian syndrome with LH levels over 35 iu/l. The ovulation rate was 90% when there was a progesterone withdrawal bleed but only 10% where there was no such bleed. Kletzky et al (1975) demonstrated the (expected) good correlation between progesterone-induced uterine bleeding and endogenous oestrogen levels. Evans (1975) demonstrated that the ovulation rate in response to clomiphene was 97% where the basal 24-h oestrogen excretion was greater than $10 \mu g/24 h$, but only 44% where it was less than this.

The underweight woman has a lower oestrogen level than the normal population and is less likely to respond to clomiphene (Knuth et al, 1977). If she gains weight, ovulation may return spontaneously or, if it does not, she may become responsive to clomiphene (Marshall and Russel-Fraser, 1971). Conception rates appear normal once ovulation is established.

Lobo et al (1982b) reported that there is a need for higher doses of clomiphene in the obese woman but that once ovulation had been achieved, obesity did not affect the ability to conceive. Similar findings were reported by Shepard et al (1979); however, 81% of patients eventually achieved ovulation if they persisted with treatment—94% of ovulating patients conceived. It has been our impression that the obese woman is less likely to become pregnant on clomiphene therapy than a woman of normal weight. Friedman and Kim (1985) report a pregnancy rate of 58% in women who are over 150% of ideal body weight compared to 70% in normal-weight women.

The factors of basal oestrogen, weight and hypothalamic or polycystic ovarian syndrome-related anovulation are clearly inter-related. It is evident that the woman with basal urinary oestrogen excretion over $10\,\mu g/24\,h$ who is of normal weight is likely to ovulate and conceive on clomiphene treatment. Women who are underweight or overweight should be encouraged to 'regress towards the mean', as this appears to improve outcome (Friedman and Kim, 1985).

## Monitoring ovulation induction with clomiphene citrate

Because of the safety and effectiveness of clomiphene there have been statements that no monitoring of these cycles is necessary (Thorneycroft, 1984). Others have based their monitoring on temperature charts, with good results (Chung, 1984; Chong et al, 1987). While agreeing that temperature charts are inexpensive, simple and harmless we do not believe that they are completely accurate. Anovulation cannot be assumed on a temperature chart that is not biphasic (Pepperell, 1984). Taymor (1987) states that there is no rational way to conduct clomiphene therapy without knowing 'that the patient is not ovulating at a particular dose level'. We believe that an assessment of ovarian response enables appropriate management to be executed.

Since the early 1960s the authors have monitored the response to treatment with clomiphene citrate at the Royal Women's Hospital by measuring the 24-h mid-luteal, urinary total oestrogen and pregnanediol (24-h O&P) excretion (Pepperell et al, 1975). If ovulation is consistently proven then monitoring can be omitted. If the pregnanediol is greater than $2\,mg/24\,h$ then ovulation is deemed to have occurred. This may also be inferred from a mid-luteal plasma progesterone level above $10\,\mu g/l$.

The advantage of the 24-h O&P is that this single measurement gives an indication of follicular response to treatment, allowing rational and effective modification of treatment without the need for other hormone or ultrasound investigations in the follicular phase. Other monitoring techniques may well be as effective, for instance, the measurement of plasma $E_2$ 7 days after the last clomiphene tablet and the measurement of progesterone 7 days after that (Adashi, 1986).

If ovulation has not occurred on the basis of the O&P result then management is decided on the basis of the oestrogen level.

1.   If the oestrogen level is less than $20\,\mu g/24\,h$, there has not been adequate follicular response and the dose of clomiphene is increased.

2.  If the oestrogen level is over 50 µg/24 h with no ovulation on the basis of the pregnanediol level, then there is follicular development but no ovulation. hCG is added at mid-cycle in the subsequent cycle.
3.  Occasionally there is follicular maturation (with an oestrogen level of 20 to 100 µg/24 h) and evidence of a deficient luteal phase or a late ovulation (with a pregnanediol level of 1.0–1.9 mg/24 h). Clomiphene is then repeated in the same dose and a second 24-h O&P may be done later in the luteal phase. If satisfactory ovulation still does not occur the dose of clomiphene is increased.

Ultrasound has become an important tool in the monitoring and treatment of difficult patients, especially where hCG is being used in addition to clomiphene. Follicular growth, measured by the diameter of the largest follicle, is greater in clomiphene-stimulated than control cycles (O'Herlihy et al, 1982; Leerentveld et al, 1985); mean follicular diameter 36 h before ovulation is 18 mm (O'Herlihy et al, 1982). Using hCG (5000 iu) when the follicle reached this diameter resulted in ovulation in 92% of cycles. In practice we have assumed a growth of 2 mm/day from the time of the sonar to evaluate the timing of hCG. This is less than the final growth rate reported in the study of O'Herlihy et al, but avoids the need for multiple scans while giving reasonable results. In general, hCG is given at follicle diameters of 18–20 mm.

Other methods of monitoring clomiphene cycles, such as temperature charts, luteal phase biopsy, serum progesterone levels, follicular phase plasma oestradiol, FSH or LH levels and serial sonar measurements, are discussed by Adashi (1986) and Hammond (1984), but have not been used in our clinic.

## How to treat the patient who is not ovulating on standard treatment

If there is no evidence of follicular development on 24-h O&P assessment as discussed above, the clomiphene dosage is increased in steps of 50 mg/day from 50 mg/day for 5 days to 250 mg/day for 5 days. If there is evidence of follicular development without ovulation hCG is added when the follicle diameter is 18–20 mm.

Where there is still no response to 250 mg/day for 5 days, incremental clomiphene is used. Currently this entails 5 days of treatment at 100 mg/day followed by 5 days at 150 mg/day. Occasionally this produces such good results that a reduction in clomiphene dose in the latter part of the treatment is required. We rarely increase the duration or dose of clomiphene above this total dose of 1250 mg over 10 days; the next step is a change to gonadotrophin or GnRH therapy.

It is clear that prolonged courses of clomiphene may induce ovulation in otherwise non-responsive patients. While initial reports concentrated on an incremental increase in clomiphene over the prolonged treatment regimen (O'Herlihy et al, 1981), subsequent reports suggest that an increase in duration of treatment may be all that is required (Lobo et al, 1982a; Garcia-Flores and Vazquez-Mendez, 1984).

The combination of clomiphene and gonadotrophins may be used in ovarian stimulation (Kemmann and Jones, 1983) but there appears to be no specific advantage in the clomiphene-resistant patient (other than reducing the human menopausal gonadotrophin (hMG) dose), with the disadvantage of a probable high rate of hyperstimulation. The regimen does have an important place however in intentional hyperstimulation for IVF.

The combination of GnRH agonist suppression of ovarian function followed by gonadotrophins has been suggested for the difficult polycystic patient (Jacobs, 1988; Lunenfeld, 1988). It is our experience and that of others (Breckwoldt et al, 1988; Coutts et al, 1988; Jacobs, 1988) that ovarian overstimulation may still occur on this regimen. A patient with polycystic ovarian syndrome treated by us developed 28 follicles of greater than 12 mm diameter, despite initial suppressive therapy with GnRH agonist for 2 weeks, followed by treatment with hMG in a dose of 300 iu/day for 5 days then 225 iu/day for 2 days.

**How to manage the patient who ovulates but does not conceive**

The great majority of pregnancies will be achieved in the first few treatment cycles. Gysler et al (1982) found that 76% of pregnancies occurred in the first two ovulatory cycles; Rust et al (1973) reported that 55% of pregnancies occur in the first two cycles and 90% in the first four. If ovulation is occurring but pregnancy has not resulted after six cycles, further action is required.

The apparent discrepancy between ovulation and pregnancy rates and the possible reasons for this have been discussed earlier. Adverse effects of clomiphene, if real, on the endometrium, oocyte or embryo cannot be dealt with other than by changing to a different treatment. Other possible fertility problems, such as poor cervical mucus or luteal phase defects, have had adjunctive treatments suggested to deal with them. The place of these various interventions will be discussed, with particular reference to our own practice.

*Ensure adequate infertility investigation*

The first and most important step in dealing with the woman who does not become pregnant while ovulating on clomiphene is to ensure that the couple have been adequately investigated. Many patients are treated before full investigations of tubal patency and the semen specimen have been done; the patient has often been given clomiphene treatment by the referring doctor. We prefer to investigate tubal patency by laparoscopy so that endometriosis can be detected earlier; however, a hysterosalpingogram is quite adequate in the first instance.

A post-coital test should also be done as part of the evaluation. If this is normal no further cervical mucus or sperm–mucus penetration tests are required. If there is apparently good mucus with an abnormal post-coital test, then full investigation of sperm–mucus interaction is indicated. If the mucus is poor it is wise to check a post-coital test or sperm–mucus inter-action study after administering 5 days of 100 µg/day of ethinyloestradiol before the test (Kroeks and Kremer, 1980). This is done to ensure that two separate problems do not coexist. Where there is abnormal sperm–mucus interaction, with or without poor mucus, we use intrauterine insemination of the husband's semen. We do this in the knowledge that the evidence for the effectiveness of this treatment is not great, although occasional successes occur (O'Herlihy et al, 1982; Alexander and Ackerman, 1987). McBain reported a pregnancy rate of 39% with intrauterine insemination where the mucus was immunologically hostile but physically normal (Kroeks and Kremer, 1980).

## Treatment with oestrogen

In women whose cervical mucus is poor at mid-cycle the question is asked: does the addition of ethinyloestradiol have a place in the clomiphene treatment cycle? O'Herlihy (1982) was unable to improve cervical mucus or pregnancy rates with the addition of ethinyloestradiol. Similarly, Chong et al (1987) were unable to improve pregnancy rates by administering ethinyl-oestradiol in cycles with poor mucus. Kemmann and Jones (1983) demonstrated a deleterious effect of clomiphene on cervical mucus in cycles treated with combined gonadotrophins and clomiphene; however, pregnancies occurred despite the poorer mucus. Given that Taubert and Dericks-Tan (1976) demonstrated that ethinyloestradiol did not interfere with ovulation induction by clomiphene, we do not have any strong objection to this treatment and it is used by some members of our clinic, usually given as 10 µg ethinyloestradiol from days 5 to 14 of the treatment cycle. This low-oestrogen dose apparently gives good clinical results (Evans, personal communication).

## The luteal phase defect

While it is known that luteal phase deficiency may occur during treatment with clomiphene, there is evidence that this problem can also be treated with clomiphene (Garcia et al, 1977; Downs and Gibson, 1983; Taymor, 1987). Huang (1986) reported no statistical difference in pregnancy rates when progesterone or clomiphene was used in the treatment of patients with luteal phase defect.

The authors have not performed luteal phase biopsies in clomiphene treatment cycles. The diagnosis of an inadequate luteal phase has been made on the basis of the luteal phase length or hormonal adequacy (as determined by urinary 24-h O&P). Treatment of a defect has been to repeat the treatment at the same clomiphene dose, but to increase dosage if the response is unimproved on the second occasion.

## The place of corticosteroid therapy

Some anovulatory patients will ovulate when given corticosteroids and some patients not ovulating on clomiphene become responsive when cortico-steroids are added. A randomized study of dexamethasone as an adjunct in clomiphene treatment showed an improved response in the dexamethasone-treated group (Daly et al, 1984). Further analysis of the results revealed that this improvement was seen in cases where the DHEAS was elevated above 200 μg/dl. Hoffman and Lobo (1985) demonstrated that clomiphene is more likely to induce ovulation where the DHEAS is below 500 μg/dl. It is likely that there is a subgroup of patients with some adrenal abnormality who may benefit from adrenal suppression.

There is a variant of congenital adrenal hyperplasia that presents late, often at the time of the menarche. The patient has an abnormal 21-hydroxylase allele but is not homozygous for the severe deficiency gene, as in the classic case. This late onset congenital adrenal hyperplasia (LOCAH), also called attenuated CAH, may be detected by stimulation with adrenocorticotrophic hormone or an analogue. The work of New et al (1983) demonstrates the overlap with values from the normal population, but with a different population mean. The 1 mg Synacthen test described by Gutai et al (1977) has been used by most gynaecological workers in this field (Rosenwaks et al, 1979; Azziz et al, 1987; Brodie and Wentz, 1987). Newmark et al (1977) reported LOCAH in 13 of 35 hirsute anovulatory women. It is clear that LOCAH can present as polycystic ovarian syndrome (Chrousos et al, 1982) and the overall incidence is probably about 10% in hirsute anovulatory women.

The authors do not believe that adrenal suppression should be given without indication; however, a case can be made for investigation of the adrenal with adrenocorticotrophic hormone stimulation tests if there is high 17OHP, high DHEAS or a failure of clomiphene treatment, whether associated with ovulation or not. It appears that cortisone acetate does not have an adverse effect on cervical mucus, although prednisolone does (Evans, personal communication); cortisone is therefore preferred in treatment and is usually administered as 25 mg at night and 12.5 mg in the morning.

*The place of other anti-oestrogens: tamoxifen*

The anti-oestrogen tamoxifen is also useful in ovulation induction (Ruiz-Velasco et al, 1979; Fukushima et al, 1982; Fukushima and Maeyama, 1983; Tajima and Fukushima, 1983; Tajima, 1984a,b). It has been our impression that this drug has less effect on cervical mucus than clomiphene citrate and this has been reported by others (Roumen et al, 1984).

Under the tutelage of Dr J. Evans we have used tamoxifen for a few cycles if 4–6 ovulatory clomiphene cycles have not resulted in pregnancy. The regimen was usually started in a dose of 10 mg twice daily (increasing to 20 mg twice daily if necessary) and given from days 3–7 of the cycle. In 38 patients without other infertility factors who ovulated after treatment with tamoxifen, there was a 23% overall pregnancy rate. Given that there had been more than four ovulatory clomiphene cycles previously in two-thirds of these women, the results are satisfactory. Seven of the nine pregnancies occurred during the first three cycles of tamoxifen treatment.

*The next step*

In the patient who is still not pregnant at this stage there is a place for treatment with gamete intrafallopian transfer (GIFT). We prefer GIFT to IVF in this situation of unexplained infertility as there appears to be a higher chance of an on-going pregnancy (Johnston, 1986; Yovich et al, 1986). Where there is a long waiting time for this treatment it will need to be considered proportionately earlier.

## A brief overview of the use of clomiphene in controlled hyperstimulation regimens

Clomiphene has been an integral part of our stimulation regimens for IVF and allied procedures. Initially clomiphene alone was used, but subsequently clomiphene in combination with (hMG) was employed because higher oocyte numbers were harvested. The development of the various regimens used at the Royal Women's Hospital, in many instances under the guidance of Dr John McBain, have been reviewed by Gronow (1985). A luteal phase defect is rare in hyperstimulation regimens using clomiphene (Gronow, 1985), although this is a common feature of gonadotrophin—only stimulation.

Yee and Vargyas (1986) and Quigley (1984) have reviewed the various clomiphene–hMG stimulation regimens used throughout the world, although it should be noted that there are very successful programmes using no clomiphene at all in their stimulation (Jones et al, 1983; Acosta et al, 1985). In general it appears that the current state of the art is that the best stimulation is the one that works best in your hands!

The current stimulation protocol used in the Reproductive Biology Unit at the Royal Women's Hospital is a sequential clomiphene–hMG regimen; this has been in use as a standard workhorse stimulation since July 1985. It was adopted after it was shown to be apparently superior to our previous one in a small cross-over study (Rogers et al, 1986). Clomiphene 100 mg/day is given for 5 days starting 10 days before the calculated mean mid-point of the last six cycles. The day after commencement of clomiphene, hMG is started in a dose of 150 iu/day (2 ampoules). This dose is adjusted in response to plasma oestradiol (or recently urinary oestrone) levels, and ceased when the plasma oestradiol ($E_2$) is over 4 nmol/l. In 848 stimulations for IVF and GIFT by the first author (McKenna), when employed as senior registrar of the Reproductive Biology Unit in 1986, a median of 6 oocytes (mean 7) were obtained after a cancellation rate before ovum pick-up of 15.4%. The median peak plasma $E_2$ was 7.1 nmol/l; the mean of the log-transformed peak $E_2$ was 7.0 nmol/l. The pregnancy rate was 18.8% overall (19% of cases had a significant male factor as a probable cause of the infertility). Spontaneous LH surges occurred in 15% of cycles but were not associated with a significant decrease in pregnancy potential.

Factors that appear intuitively obvious in hyperstimulation regimens may not be confirmed when tested. Thus, a lower dose of clomiphene may be associated with better results (Quigley et al, 1983) and an earlier start may not increase the number of oocytes (Marrs et al, 1984).

## Other uses of the anti-oestrogens

The anti-oestrogens have therapeutic applications outside the reproductive biology field. There is a place for these agents, especially tamoxifen, in the management of ovarian cancer (Quinn, 1987), breast cancer, endometrial cancer and carcinoid syndrome (particularly metastatic carcinoid tumour). The role of the anti-oestrogens in these areas is discussed later in this volume.

**Table 1.** Recommended use of anti-oestrogens.

1.  Establish that there is anovulation.
    a. Exclude hyperprolactinaemia and thyroid disease.
    b. Either initially or after 3–6 cycles:
        i. Exclude adrenal defect.
        ii. Confirm normal semen analysis.
        iii. Confirm tubal patency and exclude endometriosis.

2.  Start clomiphene at 50 mg/day from days 5–9 of natural cycle or after a progestagen withdrawal bleed (start at 25 mg/day in PCOS cases).
    a. Do not initiate a withdrawal bleed if pregnancy cannot be excluded.
    b. Assess ovarian response by hormonal evaluation: mid-luteal 24-h O&P.

| Total oestrogens (µg/24 h) | Pregnanediol (mg/24 h) | |
|---|---|---|
| <20 | <2.0 | Inadequate follicular development: increase clomiphene dose |
| >20 | >2.0 | Adequate response: repeat treatment at same dose |
| >50 | <1.0 | Follicular development without ovulation: use hCG at mid-cycle (5000 iu) when follicle diameter is 18–20 mm |
| 20–100 | 1.0–1.9 | Poor corpus luteum or late ovulation: repeat same dose. If same response increase dose (or consider hCG as above) |

3.  If there is no follicular development increase clomiphene in increments of 50 mg/day to 250 mg/day for 5 days. If still no response, use extended therapy, i.e. 100 mg/day from days 3–7 then 150 mg/day from days 8–12. If still no response ensure that there is no ovarian failure. Check FSH and LH if not done already. Then consider gonadotrophin or pulsatile GnRH therapy. In the non-responsive PCOS patient consider GnRH agonist–hMG treatment, but be aware of the risk of hyperstimulation.

4.  If patient is not pregnant after 4–6 ovulatory cycles:
    a. Investigate other causes of infertility:
        i. Tubal function.
        ii. Semen analysis and sperm antibodies.
        iii. Cervical mucus and sperm–mucus interaction.
        iv. Endometriosis.
    b. If all investigations are normal use tamoxifen for 3–6 cycles (at 10–20 mg b.d. from days 3–7 of cycle).
    c. If patient is still not pregnant consider the use of gonadotrophin therapy or GIFT.

PCOS = polycystic ovarian syndrome; 24-h O&P = 24-h total urinary oestrogen and pregnanediol; hCG = human chorionic gonadotrophin; FSH = follicle-stimulating hormone; LH = luteinizing hormone; GnRH = gonadotrophin-releasing hormone; hMG = human menopausal gonadotrophins; GIFT = gamete intrafallopian transfer.

## SUMMARY

The anti-oestrogens are important both as therapeutic agents in reproductive medicine and as tools to investigate the physiology of the oestrogen receptor and hormonal control mechanisms.

Clomiphene occupies the oestradiol receptor and, although initially stimulatory, has a net antagonistic effect as oestrogen receptors are not replenished. The major fertility-enhancing effect is to cause an increase in LH and FSH output by increasing the frequency of pulsatile output of these hormones. Many effects due to an anti-oestrogenic effect have been postulated; some, such as an adverse effect on cervical mucus, have been proven.

The clinical use of the anti-oestrogens is outlined in Table 1. In well chosen patients a rewarding pregnancy rate is obtained with minimal intervention and few important side-effects. The challenge for the reproductive biologist is successfully to manage the patient who is clomiphene-resistant, either because of failure to ovulate or failure to conceive once ovulation is induced.

## REFERENCES

Abbasi R & Hodgen GD (1986) Predicting the predisposition to osteoporosis. *Journal of the American Medical Association* **255:** 1600–1604.

Acosta AA, Bernardus RE, Jones GES et al (1985) The use of pure FSH alone or in combination for ovulation stimulation in in vitro fertilization. *Acta Europaea Fertilitatis* **16:** 81–99.

Adashi EY (1986) Clomiphene citrate initiated ovulation: a clinical update. *Seminars in Reproductive Endocrinology* **4:** 255–276.

Alexander NJ & Ackerman SA (1987) Therapeutic insemination. *Obstetrics and Gynecology Clinics of North America* **14:** 905–929.

Asch RH & Greenblatt RB (1976) Update on the safety and efficacy of clomiphene citrate as a therapeutic agent. *Journal of Reproductive Medicine* **17:** 175–180.

Ayers JWT, Drescher CW, Randolph JF, Brown A & Schneider C (1987) Abnormal gonadotrophin pulse frequency alterations induced by clomiphene citrate in 'older' women. *43rd Annual Meeting of the American Fertility Society*, p 2, abstract 4.

Azziz R, Huth J & Zacur H (1987) Reproducibility of bolus 1-24 ACTH stimulation test. *43rd Annual Meeting of the American Fertility Society*, p 85, abstract 207.

Birkenfeld A, Navot D, Levij IS et al (1986) Advanced secretory changes in the proliferative human endometrial epithelium following clomiphene citrate treatment. *Fertility and Sterility* **45:** 462–467.

Breckwoldt M, Neulen J, Wieacker P & Schellinger H (1988) Induction of ovulation by combined GnRHA/hMG/hCG treatment. *Gynaecological Endocrinology* **2 (supplement):** 68.

Brodie BL & Wentz AC (1987) Late onset congenital adrenal hyperplasia: a gynecologist's perspective. *Fertility and Sterility* **48:** 175–188.

Charles D, Klein T, Lunn SF & Loraine JA (1969) Clinical and endocrinological studies with the isomeric components of clomiphene citrate. *Journal of Obstetrics and Gynaecology of the British Commonwealth* **76:** 1100–1110.

Chong AP, Lee JL, Forte CC & Tummillo ME (1987) Identification and management of clomiphene citrate responses. *Fertility and Sterility* **48:** 941–947.

Chrousos GP, Loriaux L, Mann DL & Cutler GB (1982) Late onset 21 hydroxylase deficiency mimicking idiopathic hirsutism of polycystic ovarian disease. *Annals of Internal Medicine* **96:** 143–148.

Chung HW (1984) A rational and practical approach to clomiphene therapy. *Clinical Obstetrics and Gynecology* **27:** 953–965.

Clarke HJ, Peck EJ & Anderson JN (1974) Oestrogen receptors and antagonism of steroid hormone action. *Nature* **251**: 446–448.

Connaughton JF, Celso-Ramon G & Wallach EE (1974) Induction of ovulation with cis-clomiphene and a placebo. *Obstetrics and Gynecology* **43**: 697–701.

Corenblum B & Taylor PJ (1987) Utilization of the biochemical response to clomiphene citrate for the selection of women with hypothalamic amenorrhea who require further investigation. *Fertility and Sterility* **48**: 766–769.

Coutts JRT, Finnie S, Conaghan C, Black WP & Flemming R (1988) Combined buserelin and exogenous gonadotrophin therapy for the treatment of infertility in women with polycystic ovarian disease. *Gynaecological Endocrinology* **2 (supplement):** 71.

Cunha GR, Taguchi O, Namikawa R, Nishizuka Y & Robboy SJ (1987) Teratogenic effects of clomiphene, tamoxifen and diethylstilbestrol on the developing human female genital tract. *Human Pathology* **18**: 1132–1143.

Daly DC, Walters CA, Soto-Albors CE, Tohan N & Riddick DH (1984) A randomized study of dexamethasone in ovulation induction with clomiphene citrate. *Fertility and Sterility* **41**: 844–848.

Dodge ST, Strickler RC & Keller DW (1986) Ovulation induction with low doses of clomiphene citrate. *Obstetrics and Gynecology* **67 (supplement):** 63S–65S.

Downs KA & Gibson MG (1983) Clomiphene citrate therapy for luteal phase defect. *Fertility and Sterility* **39**: 34–38.

Evans J (1975) *The induction of ovulation in the human female*. MD thesis, University of Melbourne.

Friedman CI & Kim MH (1985) Obesity and its effect on reproductive function. *Clinical Obstetrics and Gynecology* **28**: 645–663.

Fukuma K, Fukushima T, Matso I, Mimori H & Maeyama M (1983) A graduated regimen of clomiphene citrate: its correlation to glycogen content of the endometrium and serum levels of oestradiol and progesterone in infertile patients at the midluteal phase. *Fertility and Sterility* **39**: 780–784.

Fukushima T & Maeyama M (1983) Action of tamoxifen on folliculogenesis in the menstrual cycle of infertile patients. *Fertility and Sterility* **40**: 210–214.

Fukushima T, Tajima C, Fukuma K & Maeyama M (1982) Tamoxifen in the treatment of infertility associated with luteal phase deficiency. *Fertility and Sterility* **37**: 755–761.

Gambacciani M, James HL, Williams HS et al (1987) Intrinsic pulsatility of luteinizing hormone release from the human pituitary in vitro. *Neuroendocrinology* **45**: 402–406.

Garcia J, Jones GS & Wentz A (1977) The use of clomiphene citrate. *Fertility and Sterility* **28**: 707–718.

Garcia-Flores RF & Vazquez-Mendez J (1984) Progressive doses of clomiphene in hypothalamic anovulation. *Fertility and Sterility* **42**: 543–547.

Geier A, Lunenfeld B, Pariente C et al (1987) Oestrogen receptor binding material in blood of patients after clomiphene citrate administration: determination by a radioreceptor assay. *Fertility and Sterility* **47**: 778–784.

Gronow MJ (1985) Ovarian hyperstimulation for successful in vitro fertilization and embryo transfer. *Acta Obstetrica et Gynecologica Scandinavica* **131 (supplement):** 8–10.

Grunert GM (1984) Letter. *Fertility and Sterility* **43**: 672–673.

Gutai JP, Kowarski AA & Migeon CJ (1977) The detection of the heterozygous carrier for congenital virilizing adrenal hyperplasia. *Journal of Pediatrics* **90**: 924–929.

Gysler M, March CM, Mishell DR & Bailey EJ (1982) A decade's experience with an individualized clomiphene treatment regimen including its effect on the postcoital test. *Fertility and Sterility* **37**: 161–167.

Hammond MG (1984) Monitoring techniques for improved pregnancy rates during clomiphene ovulation induction. *Fertility and Sterility* **42**: 499–509.

Hammond MG, Halme JK & Talbert LM (1983) Factors affecting the pregnancy rate in clomiphene citrate induction of ovulation. *Obstetrics and Gynecology* **62**: 196–203.

Harlap S (1976) Ovulation induction and congenital malformations. *Lancet* **ii:** 961.

Hodgen G, Kenigsburg D, Collins R & Schencken R (1985) Selection of the dominant ovarian follicle and hormonal enhancement of the natural cycle. *Annals of the New York Academy of Sciences* **442**: 23–27.

Hoffman D & Lobo RA (1985) Serum dehydroepiandrosterone sulphate and the use of clomiphene citrate in anovulatory women. *Fertility and Sterility* **43**: 196–199.

Hsueh AJW, Erickson GF & Yen SSC (1978) Sensitisation of pituitary cells to luteinising releasing hormone by clomiphene citrate in vitro. *Nature* **273:** 57–59.

Huang KE (1986) The primary treatment of luteal phase inadequacy: progesterone versus clomiphene citrate. *American Journal of Obstetrics and Gynecology* **155:** 824–828.

Insler V, Mehed H, Eden E & Lunenfeld B (1972) The cervical score. *International Journal of Gynaecology and Obstetrics* **10:** 223–228.

Jacobs HS (1988) The use of GnRH analogues in the overall management of polycystic ovarian disease. *Gynaecological Endocrinology* **2 (supplement):** 32.

Johnston WIH (1986) GIFT—cumulative results. *Clinical Reproduction and Fertility* **6:** 402–403.

Jones HW, Acosta A, Andrews MC et al (1983) The importance of the follicular phase to success and failure in in vitro fertilization. *Fertility and Sterility* **40:** 317–321.

Judd 'SJ, Alderman J, Bowden J & Michailov L (1987) Evidence against the involvement of opiate neurons in mediating the effect of clomiphene citrate on gonadotrophin-releasing hormone neurons. *Fertility and Sterility* **47:** 574–578.

Kauppila J, Janne O, Kivinen S et al (1981) Postmenopausal hormone replacement therapy with oestrogen periodically supplemented with antioestrogen. *American Journal of Obstetrics and Gynecology* **140:** 787–792.

Kemmánn E & Jones JR (1983) Sequential clomiphene citrate–menotrophin therapy for induction or enhancement of ovulation. *Fertility and Sterility* **39:** 772–779.

Kennedy JL & Adashi EY (1987) Ovulation induction. *Obstetrics and Gynecology Clinics of North America* **14:** 831–864.

Kerin JF, Liu JH, Phillipou G & Yen SC (1985) Evidence for a hypothalamic site of action of clomiphene citrate in women. *Journal of Clinical Endocrinology and Metabolism* **61:** 265–268.

Kessel B & Hsueh AJW (1987) Clomiphene citrate augments follicle-stimulating hormone induced lutenizing hormone receptor content in cultured rat granulosa cells. *Fertility and Sterility* **47:** 334–340.

Kletzky OA, Davajan V, Nakamura RM, Thorneycroft IH & Mishell DR (1975) Clinical categorization of patients with secondary amenorrhea using progesterone induced uterine bleeding and measurement of serum gonadotrophin levels. *American Journal of Obstetrics and Gynecology* **121:** 695–703.

Knuth UA, Hull MGR & Jacobs HS (1977) Amenorrhoea and loss of weight. *British Journal of Obstetrics and Gynaecology* **84:** 801–807.

Kroeks VAM & Kremer J (1980) The role of cervical factors in infertility. In Pepperell RJ, Hudson B & Wood C (eds) *The Infertile Woman,* pp 112–125. Edinburgh: Churchill Livingstone.

Kurachi K, Aono T, Minagawa J & Miyake A (1983) Congenital malformations of newborn infants after clomiphene induced ovulation. *Fertility and Sterility* **40:** 187–189.

Lamb EJ & Guderian AM (1966) Clinical effects of clomiphene in anovulation. *Obstetrics and Gynecology* **28:** 505–512.

Lamb EJ, Colliflower WW & Williams JW (1972) Endometrial histology and conception rates after clomiphene citrate. *Obstetrics and Gynecology* **39:** 389–396.

Leerentveld RA, van Gent I, van der Stoep M & Waldimiroff JW (1985) Ultrasonographic assessment of graafian follicle growth under monofollicular and multifollicular conditions in clomiphene citrate stimulated cycles. *Fertility and Sterility* **43:** 565–569.

Littman BA & Hodgen GD (1985) A comprehensive dose–response study of clomiphene citrate for enhancement of the primate ovarian/menstrual cycle. *Fertility and Sterility* **43:** 463–469.

Lobo RA, Granger LR, Davajan V & Mishell DR (1982a) An extended regimen of clomiphene citrate in women unresponsive to standard therapy. *Fertility and Sterility* **37:** 762–766.

Lobo RA, Gysler M, March CM, Goebelmann U & Mishell DR (1982b) Clinical and laboratory predictors of clomiphene response. *Fertility and Sterility* **37:** 168–173.

Lunenfeld B (1988) Indication and management of GnRH analogues in ovulation induction protocols. Abstract International symposium on GnRH analogues in cancer and human reproduction. *Gynaecological Endocrinology* **2 (supplement):** 33.

MacGregor AH, Johnson JE & Bunde CA (1968) Further clinical experience with clomiphene citrate. *Fertility and Sterility* **19:** 616–622.

MacLeod SC, Mitton DM, Parker AS & Tupper WRC (1970) Experience with induction of ovulation. *American Journal of Obstetrics and Gynecology* **108**: 814–823.

Marrs RP, Vargyas JM, Shangold GM & Yee B (1984) The effect of time of initiation of clomiphene citrate on multiple follicle development for human in vitro fertilization and embryo replacement procedures. *Fertility and Sterility* **41**: 682–685.

Marshall JC & Russel-Fraser T (1971) Amenorrhoea in anorexia nervosa: assessment and treatment with Clomiphene citrate. *British Medical Journal* **4**: 590–592.

Marut EL & Hodgen GD (1982) Antioestrogenic action of high-dose clomiphene in primates: pituitary augmentation but with ovarian attenuation. *Fertility and Sterility* **38**: 100–104.

McBain JC & Pepperell RJ (1980) Unexplained Infertility. In Pepperell RJ, Hudson B, Wood C (eds) *The Infertile Woman*, pp 164–181. Edinburgh: Churchill Livingstone.

Murphy LC & Sutherland RL (1983) Antitumor activity of clomiphene analogs in vitro: Relationship to affinity for the oestrogen receptor and another high affinity antiestrogen-binding site. *Journal of Clinical Endocrinology and Metabolism* **57**: 373–379.

New MI, Lorenzen F, Lerner AJ et al (1983) Genotyping steroid 21 hydroxylase deficiency: hormonal reference data. *Journal of Clinical Endocrinology and Metabolism* **57**: 320–326.

Newmark S, Dluhy RG, Williams GH, Pochi P & Rose LI (1977) Partial 11- and 21-hydroxylase deficiencies in hirsute women. *American Journal of Obstetrics and Gynecology* **127**: 594–598.

O'Herlihy C, Pepperell RJ, Brown JB et al (1981) Incremental clomiphene therapy: a new method for treating persistent anovulation. *Obstetrics and Gynecology* **58**: 535–542.

O'Herlihy C, Pepperell RJ & Robinson HP (1982) Ultrasound timing of human chorionic gonadotrophin administration in clomiphene stimulated cycles. *Obstetrics and Gynecology* **59**: 40–45.

Pandya G & Cohen MR (1972) The effect of cis-isomer clomiphene citrate on cervical mucus and vaginal cytology. *Journal of Reproductive Medicine* **8**: 133–138.

Pepperell RJ (1984) The investigation of infertility. In Studd J (ed.) *Progress in Obstetrics and Gynaecology*, vol. 4, pp 272–278. Edinburgh: Churchill Livingstone.

Pepperell RJ, Brown JB, Evans JH, Rennie GC & Burger HG (1975) The investigation of ovarian function by measurement of urinary oestrogen and pregnanediol excretion. *British Journal of Obstetrics and Gynaecology* **81**: 321–333.

Quigley MM (1984) The use of ovulation-inducing agents in in-vitro fertilization. *Clinical Obstetrics and Gynecology* **27**: 983–992.

Quigley MM, Maklad NF & Wolf DP (1983) Comparison of two clomiphene citrate dosage regimens for follicular recruitment in an in vitro fertilization program. *Fertility and Sterility* **40**: 178–182.

Quinn MA (1987) Hormonal therapy of ovarian cancer. In Sharp F & Soutter WP (eds) *Ovarian Cancer—The Way Ahead*, pp 383–393. London: Royal College of Obstetricians and Gynaecologists.

Rogers P, Molloy D, Healey D et al (1986) Cross-over trial of superovulation protocols from two major in vitro fertilization centres. *Fertility and Sterility* **46**: 424–431.

Rosenwaks Z, Lee PA, Jones GS, Migeon CJ & Wentz AC (1979) An attenuated form of congenital virilizing adrenal hyperplasia. *Journal of Clinical Endocrinology and Metabolism* **49**: 335–339.

Roumen FJME, Doesburg WH & Rolland R (1984) Treatment of infertile women with a deficient postcoital test with two antioestrogens: clomiphene and tamoxifen. *Fertility and Sterility* **41**: 237–243.

Ruiz-Velasco V, Rosas-Arceo J & Matute MM (1979) Chemical inducers of ovulation: comparative results. *International Journal of Fertility* **24**: 61–64.

Rust LA, Israel R & Mishell DR (1974) An individualized graduated therapeutic regimen for clomiphene citrate. *American Journal of Obstetrics and Gynecology* **120**: 785–790.

Sato F & Marrs RP (1986) The effect of pregnant mare serum gonadotrophin on mouse embryos in vivo or in vitro. *Journal of in vitro Fertilization and Embryo Transfer* **3**: 353–357.

Shepard MK, Balmaceda JP & Leija CG (1979) Relationship of weight to successful induction of ovulation with clomiphene citrate. *Fertility and Sterility* **32**: 641–645.

Skidmore J, Walpole AL & Woodburn J (1972) Effect of some triphenylethylenes on oestradiol binding in vitro to macromolecules from uterus and anterior pituitary. *Journal of Endocrinology* **52**: 289–298.

Stanger JD & Yovich JL (1985) Reduced in-vitro fertilization of human oocytes from patients with raised basal luteinizing hormone levels during the follicular phase. *British Journal of Obstetrics and Gynaecology* **92:** 385–393.

Tajima C (1984a) Tamoxifen in the treatment of infertile patients associated with inadequate luteal phase. *Fertility and Sterility* **41:** 470–472.

Tajima C (1984b) Endocrine profiles in tamoxifen-induced conception cycles. *Fertility and Sterility* **42:** 548–553.

Tajima C & Fukushima T (1983) Endocrine profiles in tamoxifen-induced ovulatory cycles. *Fertility and Sterility* **40:** 23–30.

Talbert LM (1983) Clomiphene citrate induction of ovulation. *Fertility and Sterility* **39:** 742–743.

Taubert HD & Dericks-Tan JSE (1976) High doses of oestrogens do not interfere with the ovulation inducing effect of clomiphene citrate. *Fertility and Sterility* **27:** 375–382.

Taymor ML (1987) Use and abuse of clomiphene citrate. *Fertility and Sterility* **47:** 206–207.

Testart J, Lassalle B, Belaisch-Allart J et al (1986) High pregnancy rate after early human embryo freezing. *Fertility and Sterility* **46:** 268–272.

Thatcher SS, Donachie KM, Glasier A, Hillier SG & Baird DT (1988) The effects of clomiphene citrate on the histology of human endometrium in regularly cycling women undergoing in vitro fertilisation. *Fertility and Sterility* **49:** 296–301.

Thomas A, Okamoto S, O'Shea F, McLachlan V, Besanko M & Healy DL (1987) Do raised serum luteinizing hormone levels during IVF stimulation really predict fertilization rates and clinical outcome? *Abstracts of the Sixth Annual Scientific Meeting of The Australian Fertility Society*, Sydney, 1987, p 29.

Thorneycroft IH (1984) Current status of ovulation induction with clomiphene citrate. *Fertility and Sterility* **41:** 806–808.

Van Campenhout J, Borreman ET, Wyman H & Antaki A (1973) Induction of ovulation with cisclomiphene. *American Journal of Obstetrics and Gynecology* **115:** 321–327.

Vanderhyden BC, Rouleau A, Walton EA & Armstrong DT (1986) Increased mortality during early embryonic development after in-vitro fertilization of rat oocytes. *Journal of Reproduction and Fertility* **77:** 401–409.

Yee B & Vargyas JM (1986) Multiple follicle development utilizing combinations of clomiphene citrate and human menopausal gonadotrophins. *Clinical Obstetrics and Gynecology* **29:** 141–147.

Yoshimura Y, Kitai H, Santulli R, Wright K & Wallach EE (1985) Direct ovarian effect of clomiphene citrate in the rabbit. *Fertility and Sterility* **43:** 471–476.

Yoshimura Y, Hoshi Y, Atlas SJ & Wallach EE (1986) Effect of clomiphene citrate on in vitro ovulated ova. *Fertility and Sterility* **45:** 800–804.

Yoshimura Y, Hoshi Y, Atlas SJ et al (1987a) Oestradiol reverses the limiting effects of clomiphene citrate on early embryonic development in the in vitro perfused rabbit ovary. *Fertility and Sterility* **48:** 1030–1035.

Yoshimura Y, Hosoi Y, Atlas SJ et al (1987b) Effect of the exposure of intrafollicular oocytes to clomiphene citrate on pregnancy outcome in the rabbit. *43rd Annual Meeting of the American Fertility Society*, p 21, abstract 49.

Yovich JL, Matson PL, Yovich JM, Edirisinge WR & Willcox DL (1986) Pregnancy outcome of patients conceiving after gamete manipulation. *Clinical Reproduction and Fertility* **6:** 409.

# 3

# Anti-oestrogens in the treatment of breast and gynaecological cancers

## B. J. A. FURR

Although a large number of anti-oestrogens have been described, only two, clomiphene and tamoxifen (Figure 1) have been successfully used clinically and are currently on the market. Because of its toxicity profile, clomiphene is only really used for acute therapy of anovulatory infertility. Thus, this review will inevitably concentrate on studies with Nolvadex* (tamoxifen citrate; ICI), currently the only widely used anti-oestrogen for the treatment of breast cancer which has also been evaluated in a number of gynaecological malignancies.

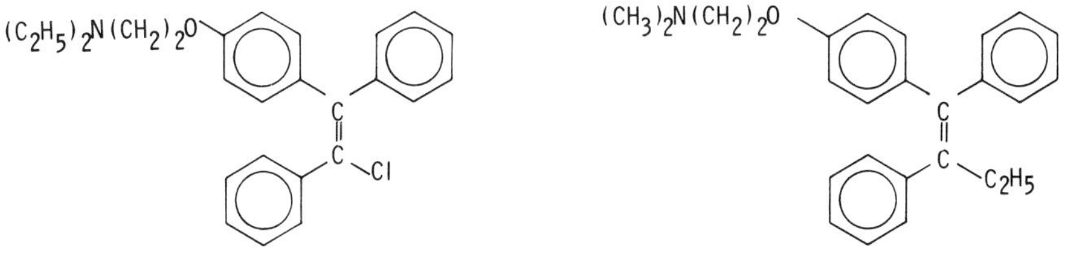

Figure 1. Structures of the clinically used anti-oestrogens clomiphene and tamoxifen.

The complex pharmacology of tamoxifen has been comprehensively reviewed by Furr and Jordan (1984). Although tamoxifen is usually described as an anti-oestrogen, it should be recognized that it can behave either as a full oestrogen agonist, a partial agonist or antagonist depending on the species, target tissue or gene product being studied. Its properties are therefore quite different from the pure anti-oestrogens recently described by Wakeling and Bowler (1987). Only time will tell whether these new compounds have improved clinical activity. Similarly, other partial agonists which are mostly close analogues of tamoxifen (droloxifene, toremifene, zindoxifene) and which are undergoing clinical trials still have to show significant clinical advantages over tamoxifen.

* Nolvadex is a trade mark, the property of ICI plc.

## BREAST CANCER

Tamoxifen has probably been more widely studied in the treatment of breast cancer than any other agent and the literature is so extensive that data summaries will be used here wherever possible.

### Advanced disease

Tamoxifen is widely accepted as the primary medical treatment for advanced breast cancer in postmenopausal women and in those premenopausal patients in whom hormonal therapy is indicated. It is estimated that the total exposure to the drug now exceeds 1.5 million patient years.

There are few good dose–response studies in respect of tamoxifen. Data summarized by Furr and Jordan (1984) suggest that there is a small improvement in response rate by increasing the dose from 20 to 40 mg/day. This is supported by two reports which show that, following progression on conventional doses of tamoxifen (20–40 mg/day), an increase in dose causes remission in some patients (Stewart et al, 1982; Watkins, 1988). However, no significant difference was found between 20 and 40 mg/day tamoxifen in a double-blind study involving 263 patients (Bratherton et al, 1984).

A mean objective response rate (complete response (CR) + partial response (PR) using International Union against Cancer (UICC) criteria) of 34% was achieved at a dose of 20–40 mg/day in 86 major clinical studies involving 5353 patients (Litherland and Jackson, 1988); disease stabilization was achieved in a further 19%, giving an overall clinical benefit of 53%. Mean or median durations of response varied from 2 to more than 24 months.

Several factors will predict the likelihood of response to tamoxifen—in particular the age of the patient, oestrogen receptor status, site of metastases and previous response to endocrine therapy (Patterson et al, 1981; Furr and Jordan, 1984). In 60 publications involving 1282 patients where response was related to age of patient, a 27% response was reported in those aged less than 50 years; in those over 70 years this increased to 43%. Indeed, many studies (Helleberg et al, 1982; Preece et al, 1982; Campbell et al, 1984; Allan et al, 1985; Bradbeer, 1985; Horgan et al, 1986; Serin et al, 1987; Gazet et al, 1988) have now suggested that tamoxifen should be used as the sole therapy for breast cancer in elderly women and the response rates obtained have been high. Although a higher response rate is seen in postmenopausal women treated with tamoxifen, a response rate of 28% was found in 302 premenopausal women in data collected from 21 studies (Jackson and Lowery, 1987). This accords very well with data from Sawka et al (1986) who found a 27% objective response rate in 74 patients.

Objective responses to tamoxifen have been obtained more often in patients with oestrogen receptor-positive tumours. However, the benefit of this anti-oestrogen is not confined to oestrogen receptor-positive tumours and clinical experience indicates that although 46% of patients with such tumours respond, up to 12% of oestrogen receptor-negative tumours show objective remission after tamoxifen therapy (Patterson et al, 1982). A number of reasons for this unexpected finding can be advanced, particularly other pharmacological properties of tamoxifen, including effects on the androgen receptor and anti-oestrogen binding site, direct cytolytic actions and effects on prostaglandin synthetase (Patterson et al, 1982). Antagonism of intracellular calcium (Lipton and Morris, 1986), calmodulin (Lam, 1984) effects at the histamine receptor (Kroeger and Brandes, 1985) and the stimulation of killer cell activity (Berry et al, 1987) have also been described and may have a role to play in tumour response. It seems unlikely that such a response rate in oestrogen receptor-negative patients could be due simply to misclassification of receptor content.

Consideration of response in relation to site of metastatic disease shows that patients with soft tissue disease have better objective responses (56%) to therapy with tamoxifen than those with dominant metastases in bone (33%) and viscera (35%) (Furr and Jordan, 1984). It should be emphasized, however, that response rates at all metastatic sites compare favourably with those obtained with other endocrine therapies. Of the responses documented for visceral metastases it appears that lung lesions respond more frequently than those in liver.

A previous response to hormonal therapy is also a good predictor of subsequent response to tamoxifen treatment (Patterson et al, 1981; Vuletic et al, 1981). Conversely, patients who respond initially to tamoxifen are more likely to have a response following subsequent endocrine therapy than those who failed to respond (Manni, 1987).

## Comparisons with other therapies

Two studies involving a total of 170 premenopausal patients have compared tamoxifen with oophorectomy: a similar rate and duration of response was found in both groups (Buchanan et al, 1986, Ingle et al, 1986). Comparisons of tamoxifen with other endocrine therapies such as oestrogens, androgens, progestogens and aromatase inhibitors have mostly concluded that the overall response rate and duration was similar; survival was no different but tamoxifen was better tolerated (Furr and Jordan, 1984). The combination of tamoxifen, either sequentially or concurrently, with other endocrine therapies has not consistently improved response rates except, perhaps, for sequential therapy with tamoxifen and progestogens; such treatment does not appear to influence survival (Furr and Jordan, 1984; Jackson and Lowery, 1987).

Since the majority of breast tumours probably comprise a mixed population of hormone-dependent and independent cells, there is a clear rationale for combination of tamoxifen and cytotoxic agents. However, results from clinical studies comparing the efficacy of cytotoxic agents with or without tamoxifen have not always shown an advantage for the combination (Kardinal et al, 1983; Furr and Jordan, 1984). Only in instances where the response to cytotoxic drugs is low does the addition of tamoxifen have a clear beneficial effect (Rose et al, 1981; Viladiu et al, 1985).

Several studies have investigated sequential use of tamoxifen treatment and cytotoxic chemotherapy (e.g. Jackson and Lowery, 1987). This approach has the advantage that the more toxic chemotherapy is reserved for later stages of the disease and it seems sensible, therefore, to advocate sequential treatment with tamoxifen as first-line therapy unless there are circumstances—such as rapidly progressing oestrogen receptor-negative anaplastic disease—in which initial combination chemotherapy is indicated.

## Side-effects

Tamoxifen is a very well tolerated drug and much of its clinical success is ascribed to its efficacy with few side-effects. At doses usually prescribed clinically (up to 40 mg/day), less than 2% of patients were withdrawn from therapy due to intolerance (Jackson and Lowery, 1987). The most common problem is nausea sometimes accompanied by vomiting; the second most frequent side-effect is hot flushes, although neither usually warrant drug withdrawal. Side-effects are very rarely life-threatening and many of the problems commonly associated with other endocrine treatments are absent. There has been a single report of a patient with encephalopathy following tamoxifen therapy (Kori and Marshall, 1982) but the significance of this isolated finding is unclear.

Hypercalcaemia has been reported to occur occasionally during the first few weeks of therapy in patients with osseous metastases. Because of the incidence of spontaneous hypercalcaemia in patients with bony metastases, especially when there is rapid tumour progression, it is difficult to interpret the association between hypercalcaemia and tamoxifen therapy. Drug-induced hypercalcaemia is clearly not a common problem. In view of the large number of patients treated in over 70 countries, the reported occurrence of only 91 cases of hypercalcaemia (Patterson et al, 1981) is small. Some workers (Arnold et al, 1979) have attributed the hypercalcaemia to a transient disease flare which often predicts a clinical response if the drug is continued or re-administered after a short period of withdrawal. It also seems possible that the hypercalcaemia may be associated with locally elevated prostaglandins, produced as the tumour cells die.

No cases of acute overdosage of tamoxifen have been reported. Four women who received between 120 and 160 mg tamoxifen twice daily for periods in excess of 17 months developed retinal and corneal changes but, remarkably, the drug was otherwise well tolerated (Kaiser-Kupfer and Lippman, 1978). In one of these patients the serum anti-oestrogen concentrations were over 1500 ng/ml—more than three times the upper limit obtained during therapy at 40 mg/day. Careful study of 19 patients who received tamoxifen at standard doses for up to 4 years showed no ocular toxicity (Beck and Mills, 1979), although there have been occasional reports that the drug has low-grade ocular toxicity (Vinding and Vestinielsen, 1983; Griffiths, 1987; Ashford et al, 1988). In these latter reports, however, it is uncertain whether the ocular lesions were due to tamoxifen since it is doubtful that they were precisely comparable to those seen in the studies of Kaiser-Kupfer and Lippman (1978).

There have been infrequent reports that tamoxifen treatment is associated with thromboembolic events (Nevasaari et al, 1978; Hendrick and

Subramanian, 1980; Lipton et al, 1984; Dahan et al, 1985). However, studies of lipoprotein clotting factors in the serum of patients being treated with tamoxifen mostly show no unfavourable changes (Jordan et al, 1987b; Onat et al, 1987; Auger and McKie, 1988; Wolter et al, 1988). However, Enck and Rios (1984) and Rieche (1986) found a small reduction in anti-thrombin III levels. As an increased incidence of thromboembolism is known to occur in patients with malignant disease, a causal relationship with tamoxifen has not been established.

Since tamoxifen is an anti-oestrogen, some concern has been expressed about the likelihood of it enhancing the loss of bone mineral content known to occur due to oestrogen withdrawal at the menopause. These fears have recently been allayed (Love et al, 1987; Wolter et al, 1988). Indeed, Wolter et al (1988) have shown that tamoxifen *reduces* loss of bone mineral content and conclude that the drug may have a protective effect similar to oestrogen. These data are in accord with the results of Citrin et al (1985) who showed that tamoxifen produced favourable 'oestrogen-like' changes in serum calcium and phosphate. An earlier paper (Gotfredsen et al, 1984) had claimed that tamoxifen caused bone loss; this was an extraordinary claim considering that bone loss was equivalent in the control and tamoxifen-treated groups!

Recently, long-term toxicity studies in rats have shown that tamoxifen induces development of hepatocellular carcinoma in some animals at a dose of 35 mg/kg daily, around 50–100 times the dose used clinically (De Waard and Wang, 1988). However, the drug was shown to be non-genotoxic, which suggests that the tumour induction is likely to be related to its complex pharmacology rather than to frank carcinogenicity. The relevance of this to man is unclear. In the same study animals receiving 20 and 35 mg/kg daily showed an increased incidence of cataracts. Whilst these findings clearly do not change the risk: benefit ratio in the treatment of confirmed malignancy, further evaluation of the implications for long-term therapy in benign diseases is required. It should be emphasized, however, that there are no reports of primary hepatic tumours in breast cancer patients receiving tamoxifen from a large number of clinical studies in which the follow-up now extends to over 10 years (I. Jackson, personal communication).

**Early breast cancer**

Since the absolute death rate from breast cancer has remained essentially unaltered for several decades, in spite of significant advances in diagnostic and primary treatment procedures (surgery and radiotherapy), it is clear that breast cancer is frequently metastatic at the time of diagnosis. This conclusion provides the rationale for adjuvant systemic therapy at the time of treatment of the primary disease.

Effective adjuvant therapy should prolong both disease-free and overall survival without a marked reduction in the quality of life of the patient. Although increase in overall survival should be the ultimate objective, too much emphasis has been placed on this parameter. Drugs with few side-effects that increase disease-free survival will be seen by the patient and her family to have significant benefit, not least of which is the psychological benefit of delay in recurrence.

In 1985, the United States National Institutes of Health convened a Consensus Development Conference to consider the role of adjuvant chemotherapy and endocrine therapy in primary breast cancer. An overview of mortality results in randomized trials in early breast cancer formed the basis of recommendations concerning its management (Lippman and Chabner, 1986). It was concluded that tamoxifen was the preferred therapy in postmenopausal women with positive nodes and positive hormone receptor levels. However, for premenopausal patients with histologically positive axillary lymph nodes and regardless of hormone receptor status, the standard treatment was considered to be adjuvant chemotherapy. The desirability of further clinical trials to elucidate the role of these treatments in other patient subgroups was emphasized.

The overview analysis involved more than 16 000 women participating in tamoxifen trials and these included a number of major studies involving substantial numbers of patients. Details of these are shown in Table 1. Hereafter, the major trials mentioned in the text refer to those shown at the top of this table.

The recommendations of the Consensus Meeting raise questions concerning the role of adjuvant tamoxifen, such as optimum duration of therapy, use in node-negative and premenopausal patients and the relevance of oestrogen receptor status of the primary tumour to treatment outcome. In addition, the desirability of co-administration of tamoxifen with cytotoxic chemotherapy has attracted much discussion. Resolution of such issues will allow the clinician to decide on the most appropriate use of tamoxifen as adjuvant treatment.

*Duration of therapy.* The optimum duration of adjuvant therapy for tamoxifen has not been determined. In most published adjuvant studies the drug has been administered for 1 or 2 years but there is evidence that longer periods of treatment may provide additional benefit. Fisher et al (1986) showed that when selected patients in the NSABP-BO9 trial were given tamoxifen alone for a third year, an improvement in disease-free and overall survival occurred compared with a group of patients who had stopped taking the drug after 2 years. These results confirm the earlier work of Tormey and Jordan (1984) who conducted a pilot study in which half the patients who had been assigned to chemotherapy plus tamoxifen for a median of 14 months went on to receive tamoxifen indefinitely. Recurrence-free survival and overall survival data favoured the long-term administration of the drug; follow-up currently exceeds 11 years. More recently, the Scottish Adjuvant Trial (1987) involved a 5-year treatment schedule with tamoxifen; this had demonstrated significant survival advantages compared with a policy of administration of the drug at first recurrence. Further data are required to determine the effects of even longer-term treatment with tamoxifen and studies presently underway, in which the drug is being given for periods of 5 years or more, should provide this information.

Table. Major trials of the adjuvant use of tamoxifen in early breast cancer.

| Trial | Case–Western Marshall et al (1987) | NSABP Fisher et al (1986) | Stockholm–Gotland Rutqvist et al (1987) | Copenhagen Palshof et al (1985) | DBCG Mouridsen et al (1986) | Christie Ribeiro and Swindell (1985) | NATO (1988) | Ludwig Goldhirsch and Gelber (1986) | The Scottish Cancer Trial (1987) | Toronto–Edmonton Meakin (1986) Pritchard et al (1987) |
|---|---|---|---|---|---|---|---|---|---|---|
| Number of evaluable patients | 311 | 1858 | 1407 | 368 | 1650 | 961 | 1131 | 629 | 1312 | 391 |
| Menopausal status | Pre Post | Pre Post | Post | Pre Post | Post | Pre Post | Pre Post | Post | Pre Post | Post |
| Age (years) | <76 | <70 | <70 | 50–79 | 50–79 | <70 | <75 | <80 | <80 | ≥50 |
| Stage | II | II, III | I, II, III | I, II, III | II, III | I, II, III | I, II | II | I, II, III | II, III |
| Tamoxifen dosage | 20 mg/b.d. 1 year | 10 mg/b.d. 2 years* | 20 mg/b.d. 2 years | 30 mg/b.d. 2 years | 30 mg/b.d. 2 years | 20 mg/b.d. 1 year | 10 mg/b.d. 2 years | 10 mg/b.d. 1 year | 20 mg/b.d. 5 years | 30 mg/b.d. 2 years |
| Study design | CMF vs tamoxifen + CMF vs CMF + tamoxifen + BCG | L-PAM+ 5FU vs L-PAM+ 5FU + tamoxifen | Favourable group: control vs tamoxifen vs tamoxifen + CMF Unfavourable group: tamoxifen + CMF vs tamoxifen + radiotherapy vs radiotherapy CMF vs radiotherapy | Premenopausal Placebo vs tamoxifen Postmenopausal Placebo vs tamoxifen vs diethylstilboestrol | Radiotherapy vs tamoxifen + radiotherapy | Premenopausal Radiation menopause vs tamoxifen Postmenopausal Control vs tamoxifen | Control vs tamoxifen | LBCS III CMFP vs P+ tamoxifen vs control LBCS IV P + tamoxifen vs control | Control vs tamoxifen | Control vs tamoxifen |
| Follow-up (months) | 78 | 72 | 53 | 78 (median) | 60 | 84 | 66 (median) | 48 | 30–96 (median duration of therapy 47) | 56 |
| Comment | ↑ in disease-free survival in tamoxifen group for oestrogen receptor-positive patients (P=0.09) | ↑ in disease-free survival for tamoxifen group (P=0.002) | ↓ recurrences in tamoxifen group (P<0.01) | ↑ in disease-free survival in postmenopausal women | ↑ recurrence-free survival for tamoxifen (P=0.0008) | Prolongation of DFI (p=0.04) and reduction in mortality (P=0.05) for tamoxifen | Prolongation of DFI (p=0.0001) and reduction in mortality (P=0.0062) for tamoxifen | ↑ in disease-free survival (p=0.0002) for endocrine treatment | Delay in relapse (p<0.0001), improvement in overall survival (P=0.002) | ↑ in disease-free survival for tamoxifen (P=0.002) |

*Some patients received treatment for 3 years.

CMF = cyclophosphamide/methotrexate/5-fluorouracil; BCG = Bacillus Calmette-Guerin; LPAM = melphalan; 5FU = 5-fluorouracil; CMFP = Cyclophosphamide/methotrexate/5-fluorouracil/prednisone; LBCS III = Ludwig Breast Cancer Study III; LBCS IV = Ludwig Breast Cancer Study IV; P = Prednisone; NSABP = National Surgical Adjuvant Breast and Bowel Project; DBCG = Danish Breast Cancer Group.

*Nodal status.* Although patients without nodal involvement at presentation generally have a good prognosis, the data available from clinical trials indicate that tamoxifen can benefit patients with node-negative breast cancer. The Stockholm–Gotland study reported statistically fewer recurrences in such a group and in both the Nolvadex Adjuvant Treatment Organisation (NATO) and Scottish studies the improvements in overall survival and disease-free survival occurred irrespective of nodal status. In the Christie trial, a beneficial effect was also recorded in patients with no lymph node involvement. These four studies have involved over 2000 patients with node-negative disease at presentation and argue strongly that the recommendation of the NIH Consensus Conference that such patients remain untreated until recurrence should be reconsidered. This view has certainly now been reached by the US National Cancer Institute which recently issued a clinical alert (Anon, 1988) stating that: 'adjuvant hormonal or cytotoxic chemotherapy can have a meaningful impact on the natural history of node negative breast cancer'.

*Premenopausal patients.* Although most of the studies investigating adjuvant use of tamoxifen alone have included postmenopausal patients, a few studies, which have involved almost 1000 premenopausal women, have also shown a treatment benefit in this group. In the NATO and Scottish trials a survival advantage was shown irrespective of menopausal status, while the Christie study noted that patients receiving either tamoxifen or an irradiation menopause had a similar survival rate. The Copenhagen trial, however, showed no significant benefit in 218 patients randomized to receive tamoxifen for 1 year compared to placebo. Increases in circulating oestradiol in premenopausal patients receiving tamoxifen have been reported (Manni et al, 1981; Jordan et al, 1987a) and it has been suggested that this may compromise effective oestrogen receptor blockade during extended periods of treatment (Jordan et al, 1987a). This possibility could be overcome by castration, which would remove the primary source of oestrogen. In these circumstances concomitant tamoxifen treatment would inhibit the effects of oestrogen derived from other sources, such as the adrenal cortex or intratumour aromatization of androgen. The use of luteinizing hormone-releasing hormone analogues, such as Zoladex* (ICI; see Furr and Milsted, 1988), to achieve a medical castration, thus removing the need for surgical intervention or the use of radiotherapy, has been advocated (Williams et al, 1986).

*Combined use of tamoxifen with cytotoxic chemotherapy.* The addition of tamoxifen to combination chemotherapy regimens has resulted in prolongation of disease-free survival compared with chemotherapy alone in some studies. The Case–Western trial showed that the addition of tamoxifen to cyclophosphamide/methotrexate/5-fluorouracil CMF significantly delayed recurrence, especially in patients with oestrogen receptor-positive tumours. The NSABP-BO9 trial also indicated that the addition of tamoxifen to combination chemotherapy produced a significant

* Zoladex is a trade mark, the property of ICI plc.

prolongation of disease-free survival. Similar results were reported from the Ludwig group, where disease-free survival was significantly longer in the patients receiving chemoendocrine therapy than in those receiving endocrine treatment with prednisone plus tamoxifen. These trials, which include over 2500 patients, have nearly all investigated the effect of chemoendocrine therapy compared with chemotherapy alone. Observations that the combination of cytotoxics and tamoxifen may have possible disadvantages compared with chemotherapy alone in premenopausal patients (Fisher et al, 1986; Dombernowsky et al, 1987) require further investigation.

*Oestrogen receptor status.* The relationship between oestrogen receptor status and response to endocrine therapy has been much debated. Although consideration of oestrogen receptor status is generally accepted as a useful predictor of response to tamoxifen in advanced disease, results in the adjuvant setting have been less clear-cut. The therapeutic efficacy of tamoxifen regarding disease-free survival was significantly correlated with oestrogen receptor status in the Ludwig, Toronto, ECOG (Tormey et al, 1986) Copenhagen and NSABP trials for postmenopausal women. In the Stockholm–Gotland study a significant increase in recurrence-free survival was noted in tamoxifen-treated patients with oestrogen receptor-rich tumours. In those with low levels of oestrogen receptor, the recurrence-free survival was slightly, but not significantly, increased. However, the NATO and Scottish trials reported that response to tamoxifen was independent of oestrogen receptor status—although in the Scottish study a gradation of response was noted, with greater survival benefit apparent in patients with higher levels of tumour oestrogen receptor, especially those greater than 100 fmol/mg protein. It is difficult to account for the discrepancies in these clinical findings, although the reliability of assay results has been questioned. A therapeutic effect of tamoxifen in patients with oestrogen receptor-negative tumours could be explained by mechanisms of action, which are not initiated by oestrogen receptor binding. Additional pharmacological properties of the drug may be relevant in this situation, as mentioned earlier.

*Tolerability of tamoxifen as adjuvant therapy.* Tamoxifen offers major advantages over chemotherapy, which causes acute toxicity in almost all patients (Henderson, 1987). When the drug has been added to cytotoxic chemotherapy regimens, increased toxicity (hot flushes, oedema) was reported in some studies but not others. In the Christie and NATO trials which involved 1–2 years treatment, tamoxifen was well tolerated: only 4% of patients were withdrawn because of side-effects. The Scottish study noted that prolonged therapy for 5 years was not associated with an increase in toxicity compared with shorter periods of treatment.

## ENDOMETRIAL CANCER

The presence of oestrogen and progesterone receptors in endometrial tumours and the fact that sex steroid hormones affect the growth and differentiation of the normal uterus provide a rationale for use of tamoxifen in the treatment of endometrial cancer. The balance of evidence suggests that tamoxifen behaves principally as an anti-oestrogen on the human uterus (Furr and Jordan, 1984) but, like oestrogen, it is capable of inducing the synthesis of uterine progesterone receptors. Litherland and Jackson (1988) have recently reviewed the accumulated data on the effect of tamoxifen on endometrial cancer. An objective response rate of 25.5% was seen in a total of 259 patients entered into 13 studies; a further 26.6% of patients had stable disease. This response rate is comparable to other endocrine therapies. Whether tamoxifen is effective in patients with tumours which have become refractory to progestogen, frequently used as first-line treatment for endometrial cancer, is controversial. Rendina et al (1984) suggested that the anti-oestrogen was effective in a proportion of such patients, whilst Edmonson et al (1986) stated categorically that it is ineffective. Certainly, there seems little advantage in combining tamoxifen with progestogens as a concurrent therapy.

The ability of tamoxifen to induce progesterone receptors in the human uterus (Furr and Jordan, 1984) has been used as a rationale for sequential therapy with tamoxifen followed by progestogens. However, Kline et al (1987) failed to show any advantage for such a regimen and the response rate was generally poor.

Perhaps surprisingly, tamoxifen does not appear to have been assessed in the treatment of vaginal or cervical cancer, although both tissues are known to be sex hormone-responsive.

## OVARIAN CANCER

Observations that around 50% of ovarian carcinomas are oestrogen receptor-positive (Bergqvist et al, 1981; Schwartz et al, 1982) prompted the evaluation of anti-oestrogen therapy. In a review of data on 346 patients from 11 studies, Litherland and Jackson (1988) reported an objective response rate of only 11.3%; a further 36.4%, however, had static disease. Although these results superficially appear disappointing, it should be emphasized that the majority of patients had been heavily pretreated and had relapsed on cytotoxic chemotherapy. It is doubtful whether better results would have been obtained in such a heavily pretreated group of breast cancer patients. More extensive studies are required to determine the precise place of tamoxifen in the treatment of ovarian cancer and trials of the drug as a primary therapy are clearly warranted.

## SUMMARY

Tamoxifen is an effective therapy for advanced breast cancer and is well tolerated. In elderly patients or in those with inoperable primary disease tamoxifen is as effective as surgery or radiotherapy. In early breast cancer tamoxifen is associated with a prolongation of disease-free and overall survival, at least in women over the age of 50 with nodal involvement. Major trials now suggest that the effectiveness of tamoxifen may, however, be independent of age, menopausal status and of nodal status, but this remains the subject of substantial controversy. These trials also suggest that longer periods of tamoxifen treatment (more than 2 years) are better than shorter treatments and, therefore, adjuvant tamoxifen until recurrence may be the final treatment of choice for such patients.

Tamoxifen is also effective in the treatment of endometrial cancer; however, there seems little advantage in combining the drug with progestogens, either concurrently or sequentially. Modest clinical benefit has been seen in patients with ovarian cancer treated with tamoxifen but the majority of patients have been heavily pretreated. Clinical trials of tamoxifen as primary therapy for this disease are warranted.

Tamoxifen has probably been the most widely studied endocrine therapy for breast cancer and the subject of some of the longest and best controlled studies. Although there is no doubt that tamoxifen is effective in adjuvant therapy of breast cancer, the precise position and duration of treatment remains to be defined unequivocally. Future use in the treatment of women at high risk of developing breast cancer—so-called prophylactic therapy—depends on improvements in risk factor determination and a continuing evaluation of the possible clinical relevance of findings in animals given long-term treatment with high doses of the drug.

## Acknowledgements

I am grateful to my colleagues Ian Jackson, Steve Litherland and Jo Diver for their help in preparing this manuscript and to Jean Appleton for patiently deciphering my writing and typing the manuscript.

## REFERENCES

Allan SG, Rodger A, Smyth JF, Leonard RCF, Chetty U & Forrest AP (1985) Tamoxifen as primary treatment of breast cancer in elderly or frail patients: a practical management. *British Medical Journal* **290:** 358.

Anon (1988) *The Clinical Cancer Letter* **11:** 1–4.

Arnold DJ, Markham MJ & Hacker S (1979) Tamoxifen flare. *Journal of the American Medical Association* **241:** 2506.

Ashford AR, Donev I, Tiwari RP & Garrett TJ (1988) Reversible ocular toxicity related to tamoxifen therapy. *Cancer* **61:** 33–35.

Auger MJ & McKie MJ (1988) Effect of tamoxifen on blood coagulation. *Cancer* **61:** 1316–1319.

Beck M & Mills PV (1979) Ocular assessment of patients treated with tamoxifen. *Cancer Treatment Reports* **63:** 1833–1834.

Bergqvist A, Kullander S & Thorell J (1981) A study of estrogen and progesterone cytosol receptor concentration in benign and malignant ovarian tumors and a review of malignant ovarian tumours treated with medroxyprogesterone acetate. *Acta Obstetrica et Gynecologica Scandinavica* **supplement 101:** 75–81.

Berry J, Green BJ & Matheson DS (1987) Modulation of natural killer cell activity by tamoxifen in stage 1 postmenopausal breast cancer. *European Journal of Cancer and Clinical Oncology* **23:** 517–520.

Bradbeer JW (1985) Treatment of primary breast cancer in the elderly with Nolvadex alone. *Reviews on Endocrine-related Cancer* **supplement 16:** 39–42.

Bratherton DG, Brown CH, Buchanan R et al (1984) A comparison of two doses of tamoxifen (Nolvadex) in postmenopausal women with advanced breast cancer: 10 mg b.d. versus 20 mg b.d. *British Journal of Cancer* **50**: 199–205.

Buchanan RB, Blamey RW, Durrant KR et al (1986) A randomised comparison of tamoxifen with surgical oophorectomy in premenopausal patients with advanced breast cancer. *Journal of Clinical Oncology* **4**: 1326–1330.

Campbell FE, Morgan DAL, Bishop HM et al (1984) The management of locally advanced carcinoma of the breast by Nolvadex (tamoxifen): a pilot study. *Clinical Oncology* **10**: 111–115.

Citrin DL, Ingle J, O'Fallon J et al (1985) Effect of diethylstilbestrol (DES) and tamoxifen (TAM) on serum (Se) calcium (Ca) and phosphate ($PO_4$) in metastatic breast cancer (BC). In *Proceedings of Breast Cancer Research Conference*. London: Imperial Cancer Research Fund, abstract C–15, p 219.

Dahan R, Espie M, Mignot L, Houlbert D & Chanu B (1985) Tamoxifen and arterial thrombosis. *Lancet* **i**: 638.

De Waard F & Wang DY (1988) Epidemiology and prevention: workshop report. *European Journal of Cancer and Clinical Oncology* **24**: 45–48.

Dombernowsky P, Mouridsen HT, Brincker H et al (1987) Adjuvant treatment with CMF + radiotherapy (RT) versus CMF versus CMF + tamoxifen (TAM) in pre and post-menopausal high risk breast cancer patients. In *Fourth EORTC Breast Cancer Working Conference*, abstract C2D 14.

Edmonson JH, Krook JE, Hilton JF et al (1986) Ineffectiveness of tamoxifen in advanced endometrial carcinoma after failure of progestin treatment. *Cancer Treatment Reports* **70**: 1019–1020.

Enck RE & Rios CN (1984) Tamoxifen treatment of metastatic breast cancer and antithrombin III levels. *Cancer* **53**: 2607–2609.

Fisher B, Redmond C, Brown A et al (1986) Adjuvant chemotherapy with and without tamoxifen in the treatment of primary breast cancer: 5-year results from the National Surgical Adjuvant Breast and Bowel Project Trial. *Journal of Clinical Oncology* **4**: 459–471.

Furr BJA & Jordan VC (1984) The pharmacology and clinical uses of tamoxifen. *Pharmacology and Therapeutics* **25**: 127–205.

Furr BJA & Milsted RAV (1988) LH-RH analogues in cancer treatment. In Stoll BA (ed.) *Endocrine Management of Cancer. 2. Contemporary Therapy*, pp 16–29. Basel: Karger.

Gazet J-C, Forad HT, Bland JM, Markopoulos Ch, Coombes RC & Dixon RC (1988) Prospective randomised trial of tamoxifen versus surgery in elderly patients with breast cancer. *Lancet* **i**: 679–681.

Goldhirsch A & Gelber R (1986) Adjuvant treatment for early breast cancer: the Ludwig breast cancer studies. *National Cancer Institute Monographs* **1**: 55–70.

Gotfredsen A, Christiansen C & Palshof T (1984) The effect of tamoxifen on bone mineral content in premenopausal women with breast cancer. *Cancer* **53**: 853–857.

Griffiths MFP (1987) Tamoxifen retinopathy at low dosage. *American Journal of Ophthalmology* **104**: 185–186.

Helleberg A, Lundgren B, Norin T & Sander S (1982) Treatment of early localised breast cancer in elderly patients by tamoxifen. *British Journal of Radiology* **55**: 511–515.

Henderson IC (1987) Adjuvant systemic therapy for early breast cancer. *Current Problems in Cancer* **11**: 128–207.

Hendrick A & Subramanian VP (1980) Tamoxifen and thromboembolism. *Journal of the American Medical Association* **243**: 514–515.

Horgan K, Mansel RE & Webster DJT (1986) Tamoxifen as sole therapy for localised breast cancer. *European Journal of Cancer and Clinical Oncology* **22**: 114.

Ingle JN, Krook JE, Green SJ et al (1986) Randomised trial of bilateral oophorectomy versus tamoxifen in premenopausal women with metastatic breast cancer. *Journal of Clinical Oncology* **4**: 178–185.

Jackson IM & Lowery C (1987) Clinical uses of antioestrogens. In Furr BJA & Wakeling AE (eds) *Pharmacology and Clinical Uses of Inhibitors of Hormone Secretion and Action*, pp 87–105. London: Baillière Tindall.

Jordan VC, Fritz NF & Tormey DC (1987a) Endocrine effects of adjuvant chemotherapy and long-term tamoxifen administration on node positive patients with breast cancer. *Cancer Research* **47**: 624–630.

Jordan VC, Fritz NF & Tormey DC (1987b) Long term adjuvant therapy with tamoxifen. Effects on sex hormone binding globulin and antithrombin III. *Cancer Research* **47**: 4517–4519.

Kaiser-Kupfer MI & Lippman ME (1978) Tamoxifen retinopathy. *Cancer Treatment Reports* **62**: 315–320.

Kardinal CG, Perry MC, Weinberg G, Wood W, Ginsberg S & Raju RN (1983) Chemo-endocrine therapy vs chemotherapy alone for advanced breast cancer in postmenopausal women: preliminary report of a randomised study. *Breast Cancer Research and Treatment* **3**: 365–372.

Kline RC, Freedman RS, Jones LA & Atkinson EN (1987) The treatment of recurrent or metastatic poorly-differentiated adenocarcinoma of the endometrium with tamoxifen and medroxyprogesterone acetate. *Cancer Treatment Reports* **71**: 327–328.

Kori SH & Marshall J (1982) Tamoxifen-induced encephalopathy. *Neurology* **32**: A72–A73.

Kroeger EA & Brandes LJ (1985) Evidence that tamoxifen is a histamine antagonist. *Biochemical and Biophysical Research Communications* **131**: 750–755.

Lam HYP (1984) Tamoxifen is a calmodulin antagonist in the activation of CAMP phospho-diesterase. *Biochemical and Biophysical Research Communications* **118**: 27–32.

Lippman ME & Chabner BA (1986) Editorial overview. *National Cancer Institute Monographs* **1**: 5–10.

Lipton A & Morris ID (1986) Calcium antagonism by the antioestrogen tamoxifen. *Cancer Chemotherapy and Pharmacology* **18**: 17–20.

Lipton A, Harvey HA & Hamilton RW (1984) Venous thrombosis as a side-effect of tamoxifen treatment. *Cancer Treatment Reports* **68**: 887–889.

Litherland S & Jackson I (1988) Antioestrogens in the management of hormone-dependent cancer: a review. *Cancer Treatment Reviews* (in press).

Love RR, Mazess RB, Tormey DC, Rasmussen P & Jordan VC (1987) Bone mineral density (BMD) in women with breast cancer treated with tamoxifen for two years. *Breast Cancer Research Treatment* **10**: 112.

Manni A (1987) Tamoxifen therapy of metastatic breast cancer. *Journal of Laboratory and Clinical Medicine* **109**: 290–299.

Manni A, Arafah B & Pearson OH (1981) Changes in endocrine status following antioestrogen administration to premenopausal and postmenopausal women. In Sutherland RL & Jordan VC (eds) *Non-Steroidal Antioestrogens*, pp 435–452. Sydney: Academic Press.

Marshall JS, Gordon NH, Hubay CA & Pearson OH (1987) Assessment of tamoxifen as adjuvant therapy in stage II breast cancer: a long-term follow-up. *Journal of Laboratory and Clinical Medicine* **109**: 300–307.

Meakin JW (1986) Review of Canadian trials of adjuvant endocrine therapy for breast cancer. *National Cancer Institute Monographs* **1**: 111–113.

Mouridsen HT, Andersen AP, Brincker H, Dombernowsky P, Rose C & Andersen KW (1986) Adjuvant tamoxifen in postmenopausal high-risk breast cancer patients: present status of Danish breast cancer cooperative group trials. *National Cancer Institute Monographs* **1**: 115–118.

Nevasaari K, Heikkinen M & Taskinen PJ (1978) Tamoxifen and thrombosis. *Lancet* **ii**: 946–947.

Nolvadex Adjuvant Trial Organisation (1988) Controlled trial of tamoxifen as a single adjuvant agent in the management of early breast cancer. *British Journal of Cancer* **57**: 608–611.

Onat H, Inceman S, Bilge N, Dincol K, Tore G & Topuz E (1987) Effect of tamoxifen on antithrombin III activation in breast cancer patients. *Proceedings of the 15th International Congress of Chemotherapy, Istanbul* **3**: 279–281.

Palshof T, Carstensen B, Mouridsen HT & Dombernowsky P (1985) Adjuvant endocrine therapy in pre- and postmenopausal women with operable breast cancer. *Reviews on Endocrinology Related Cancer* **17**: 43–50.

Patterson JS, Edwards DG & Battersby LA (1981) A review of the international clinical experience with tamoxifen. *Japanese Journal of Cancer Clinics* **supplement**: 157–183.

Patterson J, Furr B, Wakeling A & Battersby L (1982) The biology and physiology of Nolvadex (tamoxifen) in the treatment of breast cancer. *Breast Cancer Research and Treatment* **2**: 363–374.

Preece PE, Wood RAB, Mackie CR & Cuschieri A (1982) Tamoxifen as initial sole treatment of localised breast cancer in elderly women: a pilot study. *British Medical Journal* **284:** 869–870.

Pritchard KI, Meakin JW, Boyd N et al (1987) Adjuvant tamoxifen in postmenopausal women with axillary node positive breast cancer: an update. *Proceedings of the Vth International Conference on Adjuvant Therapy of Cancer, Tucson, USA* abstract 57.

Rendina GM, Donadio C, Fabri M, Mazzoni P & Nazzicone P (1984) Tamoxifen and medroxyprogesterone therapy for advanced endometrial carcinoma. *European Journal of Obstetrics, Gynecology and Reproductive Biology* **17:** 285–291.

Ribeiro G & Swindell R (1985) The Christie Hospital tamoxifen Nolvadex adjuvant trial for operable breast carcinoma—seven year results. *European Journal of Cancer and Clinical Oncology* **21:** 897–900.

Rieche K (1986) Influence of tamoxifen and aminoglutethimide on antithrombin III levels in patients with metastatic breast cancer. *Haemostasis* **16 (supplement 5):** abstract 110.

Rose C, Mouridsen HT & Palshof T (1981) Combination of tamoxifen with cytotoxic or endocrine therapy. *Reviews on Endocrine Related Cancer* **9:** 455–471.

Rutqvist LE, Cedermark B, Glas U et al (1987) The Stockholm trial on adjuvant tamoxifen in early breast cancer. Correlation between estrogen receptor level and treatment effect. *Breast Cancer Research and Treatment* **10:** 255–266.

Sawka CA, Pritchard KI, Paterson AHG et al (1986) Role and mechanism of action of tamoxifen in premenopausal women with metastatic breast carcinoma. *Cancer Research* **46:** 3152–3156.

Schwartz PE, Keating G, MacClusky N, Naftolin F & Eisenfeld A (1982) Tamoxifen therapy for advanced ovarian cancer. *Obstetrics and Gynecology* **59:** 583–588.

Serin D, Martin P, Bigi N, Martin D & Reboul F (1987) Cancer du sein chez la femme âgée: traitement initial par le tamoxifène. Résultats preliminaires. *Contraception–Fertilité–Sexualité* **15:** 1091–1093.

Stewart JF, Minton MJ & Rubens RD (1982) Trial of tamoxifen at a dose of 40 mg daily after disease progression during tamoxifen therapy at a dose of 20 mg daily. *Cancer Treatment Reports* **66:** 1445–1446.

The Scottish Cancer Trial (1987) Adjuvant tamoxifen in the management of operable breast cancer. *Lancet* **ii:** 171–175.

Tormey DC & Jordan VC (1984) Long term tamoxifen adjuvant therapy in node-positive breast cancer: a metabolic and pilot clinical study. *Breast Cancer Research and Treatment* **4:** 297–302.

Tormey DC, Gray R, Taylor SG, Knuiman M, Olson JE & Cummings FJ (1986) Postoperative chemotherapy and chemohormonal therapy in women with node-positive breast cancer. *National Cancer Institute Monographs* **1:** 75–80.

Viladiu P, Alonso MC, Avella A et al (1985) Chemotherapy versus chemotherapy plus hormone therapy in postmenopausal advanced breast cancer patients. A randomised trial (tamoxifen, cyclophosphamide, methotrexate, 5-fluorouracil, medroxyprogesterone, adriamycin, vincristine). *Cancer* **56:** 2745–2750.

Vinding T & Vestinielsen N (1983) Retinopathy caused by treatment with tamoxifen in low dosage. *Acta Ophthalmologica* **61:** 45–50.

Vuletic L, Bugarski M, Boberic J, Milosauljevic A & Naumovic P (1981) Treatment of advanced breast cancer with tamoxifen: a report of 50 cases. *Reviews on Endocrine Related Cancer* **9:** 533–545.

Wakeling AE & Bowler J (1987) Steroidal pure antioestrogens. *Journal of Endocrinology* **112:** R7–R10.

Watkins SM (1988) The value of high dose tamoxifen in postmenopausal breast cancer patients progressing on standard doses: a pilot study. *British Journal of Cancer* **57:** 320–321.

Williams MR, Walker KJ, Turkes A, Blamey RW & Nicholson RI (1986) The use of an LHRH agonist (ICI 118,630, Zoladex) in advanced premenopausal breast cancer. *British Journal of Cancer* **53:** 629–636.

Wolter J, Ryan WG, Subbiah PV & Bagdade JD (1988) Apparent beneficial effects of tamoxifen on serum lipoprotein subfractions and bone mineral content in patients with breast cancer. *Proceedings of the American Society of Clinical Oncology, New Orleans*, abstract 34.

# 4

## Anti-androgens in gynaecological practice

M. J. REED
S. FRANKS

### INTRODUCTION

Anti-androgens are used in gynaecology in the treatment of women with symptoms arising from the action of androgens on the skin. These conditions, which include acne, seborrhoea and hirsutism, are usually benign, but they are a cause of considerable distress to women and medical therapy is desirable.

Androgens are naturally occurring steroids containing 19 carbon atoms. Androgens are defined as compounds which maintain the male reproductive tract but in addition have general anabolic effects. In women their role is less apparent although androgens influence hair growth and muscle mass. In women in whom androgen production is increased, as the result of pathological overproduction, the effects of androgens become more obvious with the development of mild forms of virilization such as acne, seborrhoea or mild hirsutism. In many patients with this clinical picture the presence of polycystic ovaries (PCO) can usually be demonstrated using biochemical and ultrasonographic techniques (Franks et al, 1985). More severe virilization, e.g. temporal hair recession or increased muscle mass, may also occur as a result of benign conditions such as PCO but in such cases the presence of an androgen-secreting tumour must be excluded before considering the use of anti-androgens.

In order to appreciate the effects that anti-androgens can have on the synthesis, availability and action of androgens, it is necessary to have an understanding of androgen physiology in normal women.

### Sources of androgens in women

The biologically active androgens found in the circulation are testosterone and dihydrotestosterone (DHT). Testosterone is secreted by the ovaries and adrenal cortex, in response to the appropriate hypothalamic–pituitary signal, and this accounts for 50% of the testosterone produced by normal women (Vermeulen, 1979). The other major source of testosterone in women arises from the peripheral conversion of androstenedione which is also secreted by the ovaries and adrenals. Therefore all circulating testosterone is derived directly or indirectly by secretion of androgen by ovary and adrenal. DHT is not secreted directly by adrenal or ovary but arises from the conversion of testosterone in target tissues such as the skin.

### Transport of androgens in blood

Androgens such as testosterone and DHT circulate in the blood in a free, non-protein-bound state, bound to albumin or to a specific plasma-binding protein—sex-hormone-binding globulin (SHBG) (Anderson, 1974). SHBG binds testosterone with a high affinity but low capacity, in contrast to albumin which binds these steroids with a low affinity but high capacity. In normal women only about 1% testosterone is present in a free state with 30 and 66% bound to albumin and SHBG respectively (Dunn et al, 1981). It has generally been considered that only the free steroid fraction is able to diffuse across cell membranes and interact with receptors and that this, therefore, represents the biologically active steroid fraction in blood (Giorgi, 1980). However, the free steroid concept has recently been challenged. Pardridge and Mietus (1979) have presented experimental evidence which suggests that the albumin-bound steroid fraction may, by dissociation, be available to some tissues. More recently, Siiteri et al (1982) have suggested that the SHBG-bound steroid fraction may, by some as yet undefined mechanism, be involved in the entry of steroids into target tissues.

### Mechanism of androgen action

The ability of testosterone to produce an androgenic response in tissues is dependent upon, firstly, the presence of intracellular receptors which bind androgens with high affinity (Anderson and Liao, 1968) and secondly, in some tissues the conversion of testosterone to DHT by the $5\alpha$-reductase enzyme (Bruchovsky and Wilson, 1968).

### Metabolism of androgens in skin

In tissue such as skin where testosterone is converted to DHT, this steroid is further metabolized by a number of different enzymes. There is currently considerable interest in measurements of serum levels of a metabolite of DHT, $3\alpha$-androstanediol-glucuronide (Adiol-G) because such measurements may provide an index of peripheral androgen metabolism (Horton et al, 1982). However, the pathway by which Adiol-G is formed is not yet clear, i.e. whether DHT is converted to androstanediol and then to Adiol-G or whether DHT is conjugated with glucuronic acid before conversion to Adiol-G.

### Origin of excess androgen production in women with clinical symptoms of androgen excess

Kirschner et al (1976) demonstrated that the production rate of testosterone is related to the degree of virilization in women. However, the source of increased androgen production in women with conditions such as mild hirsutism remains controversial. As previously discussed, a common cause of hyperandrogenization in women is the PCO syndrome. Measurement of androgen concentrations in blood from the ovarian and adrenal veins of women with PCO has produced conflicting evidence, with both the ovary (Kirschner and Jacobs, 1971) and adrenal (Stahl et al, 1973) being implicated as the source of excess androgen production. Selective inhibition and stimulation of the ovaries and adrenals have been used in an attempt to locate the source of excess androgen production, but this approach has failed to give clear-cut results (Goldzieher et al, 1978). In an attempt to examine this problem we have measured in normal women and hirsute women with PCO serum levels of 11β-hydroxyandrostenedione (11β-OHA), a steroid thought to be synthesized only in the adrenal gland. Although no difference in serum 11β-OHA levels was detected between normal subjects and patients with PCO (Figure 1), the ratio of androstenedione : 11β-OHA was considerably

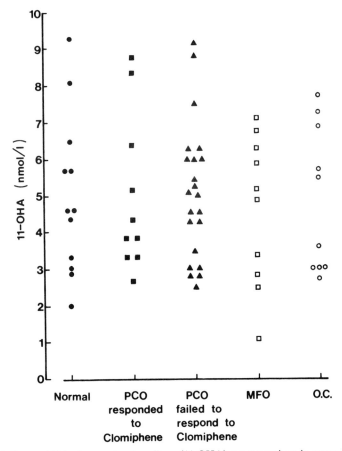

**Figure 1.** Serum 11β-hydroxyandrostenedione (11-OHA) concentrations in normal women, women with polycystic (PCO) or multifollicular ovaries (MFO) or receiving oral contraceptives (O.C.). From Polson et al (1988), with permission.

higher in women with PCO (Table 1), suggesting that the ovary is the major source of increased androgen production in these women (Polson et al, 1988).

**Table 1.** Concentrations of androstenedione (A) and 11β-hydroxyandrostenedione (11β-OHA) and ratio of A:11β-OHA in normal women and women with polycystic ovaries (PCO).

|        | A (nmol/l)    | 11β-OHA (nmol/l) | A:11β-OHA    |
|--------|---------------|------------------|--------------|
| Normal | 5.6 ± 1.7     | 5.0 ± 2.3        | 1.1 ± 0.5    |
| PCO    | 9.8 ± 3.1*    | 5.0 ± 2.1        | 2.0 ± 0.7*   |

* $P < 0.001$.

## Markers of peripheral androgen metabolism

There is currently considerable interest in establishing which androgen or androgen metabolite provides the most reliable index of peripheral androgen metabolism. This interest is stimulated by a desire to be able to differentiate on a biochemical basis hirsute from non-hirsute women. Such a marker would also be of use in monitoring the response to therapy in hirsute women. Measurements of plasma levels of testosterone, DHT or androstanediol have generally failed to discriminate between hirsute and non-hirsute women. Mean concentrations of these hormones are obviously significantly higher in hirsute compared with non-hirsute women with normal ovaries but there is too much overlap in values between the groups for these indices to be clinically useful (Baxendale et al, 1982, 1983). The ability to measure directly the free testosterone concentration in serum (Cheng et al, 1986) led us to evaluate the use of such measurements in normal and hirsute women. As previously reported for total levels of testosterone in plasma, we found that there was a considerable overlap between normal and hirsute women (Figure 2). We have also measured serum Adiol-G levels in normal and hirsute women (Figure 3). Our findings have failed to confirm the value of such measurements as a marker of peripheral androgen metabolism (Reed et al, 1986). However, our preliminary studies have shown that serum levels of another and quantitatively important androgen conjugate, androsterone glucuronide (Scanlon et al, 1987), may discriminate more clearly between normal and hirsute women (Figure 4).

From this brief review it is apparent that the clinical effects of hyper-androgenization in women may result from an increase in androgen production, a decrease in the level of SHBG, or changes in the sensitivity of tissues such as skin to androgens, which in turn may reflect increased peripheral metabolism of testosterone and androstenedione to its more potent 5α-reduced metabolite.

## ANTI-ANDROGENS

Dorfman (1970) defined an anti-androgen as a substance which prevents

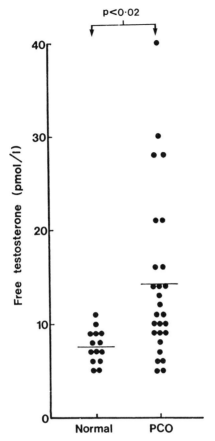

**Figure 2.** Serum free testosterone concentration in normal women and women with polycystic ovaries (PCO).

androgens from exerting their activity in target tissues at the level of the intracellular receptor. This definition would therefore exclude compounds which inhibited glandular steroidogenesis or the secretion of pituitary hormones. It is apparent, however, that the anti-androgens currently used in gynaecology do exert part of their beneficial effects by mechanisms other than by interference with the action of androgens at the cellular level. In a recent review, Biffighandi et al (1984) listed the currently known anti-androgens as: cyproterone acetate, spironolactone, RU-2956, megestrol acetate and medrogesterone. In addition to these steroidal anti-androgens, three non-steroidal compounds (stilboestrol, flutamide and cimetidine) are known to have anti-androgenic properties. So far only cyproterone acetate and spironolactone have been widely used in gynaecology. The structure of these compounds is shown in Figure 5. The use of anti-androgens in gynaecological disorders has been reviewed by Jeffcoate (1982) and Horton and Lobo (1986).

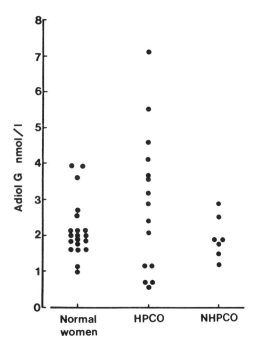

**Figure 3.** Serum androstanediol glucuronide (Adiol-G) concentrations in normal women and hirsute (HPCO) and non-hirsute (NHPCO) women with polycystic ovaries. From Scanlon et al (1988), with permission.

## Cyproterone acetate

The anti-androgen cyproterone acetate (CPA) was first used clinically by Hammerstein and Cupceancu (1969). CPA acts not only by blocking the action of androgens at the cellular level but also has strong progestational properties, resulting in the inhibition of gonadotrophin release (Giusti et al, 1977). CPA is administered in a reverse sequential regimen originally devised by Hammerstein et al (1975). For this CPA (100 mg) is administered on days 5–14 of the menstrual cycle with ethinyloestradiol (50 µg) being given throughout the cycle to maintain control of vaginal bleeding and contraception. The development of specific radioimmunoassays for CPA has shown that significant levels of CPA remain in the circulation for up to 2 weeks after the ingestion of the last tablet. In addition to the high (100 mg) dosage regimen, an oral contraceptive (o.c.) formulation containing CPA (2 mg) and ethinyloestradiol (35 µg) is also available. The response to this lower dosage of CPA is about 50% in women with mild and moderate forms of hirsutism, whereas up to 70% of women show a good response to the higher dose of CPA (Hammerstein et al, 1983).

While it is now established that treatment with CPA is an effective form of therapy for hirsutism, the form of therapy required to maintain the initial response is not clear. Up to 70% of treated patients show a marked relapse upon cessation of CPA therapy (Zielske et al, 1971; Underhill and Dewhurst, 1979). The use of lower doses of CPA to maintain the initial response has been investigated (Holdaway et al, 1985). After treatment with the 100 mg CPA regimen patients received either 25 mg CPA plus the o.c. formulation or a placebo plus the o.c. formulation. Both maintenance schedules were effective in preventing relapse after cessation of the high dosage of CPA.

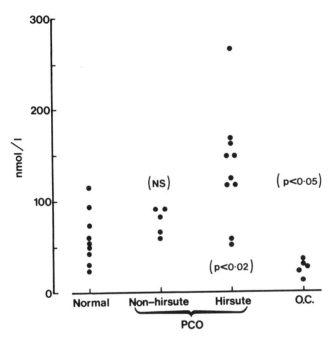

**Figure 4.** Serum androsterone glucuronide concentrations in normal women, in non-hirsute and hirsute women with polycystic ovaries (PCO) and women receiving oral contraceptive (O.C.) therapy.

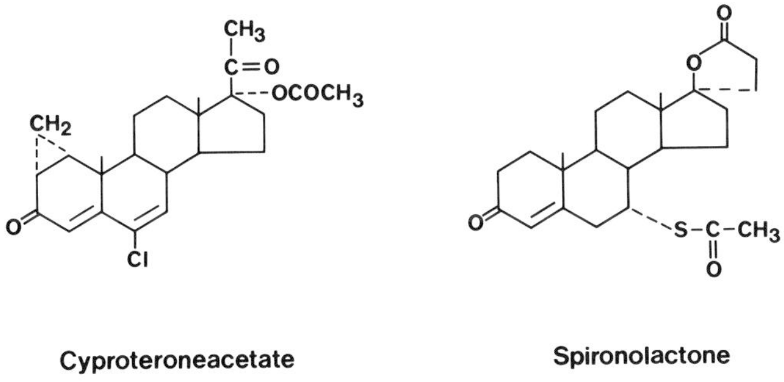

Cyproteroneacetate             Spironolactone

**Figure 5.** Structure of anti-androgens.

Although the primary action of CPA is to inhibit the association of androgens with their receptors there is good evidence that CPA also acts via other mechanisms. Using cultured pubic skin fibroblasts, Mowszowicz et al (1983) demonstrated CPA ($2 \times 10^{-6}$ mol/l) prevented the stimulation of 5$\alpha$-reductase activity by $10^{-7}$ mol/l DHT.

As CPA has progestational properties and is co-administered with oestrogen, an effect on glandular steroidogenesis and circulating free androgen levels is also likely to play a part in obtaining the clinical response associated with the reverse sequential regimen. The effect of CPA on plasma androgen levels is controversial with some (Ismail et al, 1974; Barnes et al, 1975) but not all studies (Frohlich et al, 1977; Lunnell et al, 1982) reporting a decrease in circulating androgen levels. Rubens (1984) found that plasma levels of testosterone, androstenedione and DHT decreased by 25–64%. Concurrent administration of oestrogen resulted in a 400% increase in SHBG levels, leading to a marked (70%) decrease in the calculated free testosterone concentration. Thus this treatment regimen is effective biochemically in reducing hyperandrogenism.

Although treatment with CPA is acknowledged to be effective in the treatment of hirsutism, this is usually a benign condition, and to be acceptable as a mode of treatment side-effects must be minimal. Several groups have reported on side-effects associated with the use of CPA, with the most serious suggestion being the possibility that treatment with CPA results in suppression of adrenal function. High doses of CPA can cause suppression of adrenal function in animals (Girard et al, 1978) and suppression may occur in children treated with CPA for precocious puberty (Stivel et al, 1982). In 16 adult female patients who had been treated with CPA for longer than 1 year, Hayne et al (1982) found some evidence of reduced basal cortisol output in 25% of patients, although the ability of the pituitary–adrenal axis to respond to stress remained. Results from two other investigations, however, failed to find any evidence that women treated with long-term CPA had depressed secretion of cortisol (Chapman et al, 1982; Holdaway et al, 1983). Other side-effects associated with the use of CPA include fatigue, a decrease in libido and evidence of weight gain (Hammerstein et al, 1983). Side-effects produced by the high and low (o.c.) form of CPA therapy were compared by Belisle and Love (1986). The incidence of progestational effects such as breast tenderness, amenorrhoea and weight gain were greater in women receiving the high doses of CPA whilst the occurrence of other side-effects was similar for both groups of women. The reversed sequential regimen of CPA therapy is also associated with reduced fasting plasma glucose and raised fasting plasma insulin levels. However, the elevation of insulin levels does not occur during the phase of treatment with ethinyloestradiol alone (Seed et al, 1984). There is also evidence that the lipoprotein profile may be changed unfavourably by CPA and ethinyloestradiol with a decrease, albeit a slight one, in high-density lipoprotein$_2$ concentrations (Wynn et al, 1986). There is one report of a case of pulmonary embolism developing in a woman with acne shortly after starting treatment for hirsutism with the o.c. preparation of CPA (Poran et al, 1986).

## Spironolactone

The anti-androgenic effect of spironolactone, an aldosterone antagonist, was first demonstrated in animals by Jones and Woodbury (1964). In the female the finding of menstrual irregularities in patients treated for hypertension led to the first clinical trial for the use of spironolactone in the treatment of female hirsutism (Boisselle and Tremblay, 1976).

The mechanism by which spironolactone acts is complex. In addition to competing for binding to the androgen receptor (Boisselle et al, 1979), spironolactone or its active metabolite canrenone (Boisselle et al, 1979) inhibits glandular steroidogenesis by decreasing the levels of microsomal cytochrome P450-dependent enzymes (Menhard et al, 1976). This results in decreased activity of 11β-, 17- and 21-hydroxylase enzymes. An increase in the conversion of androgens to oestrogens also occurs (Rose et al, 1977).

Several studies have shown that spironolactone is effective in the treatment of hirsutism (Boisselle and Tremblay, 1979; Shapiro and Evron, 1980; Milewicz et al, 1983; Lobo et al, 1985), although variable effects on plasma androgen levels have been reported (Evans and Burke, 1986; Young et al, 1987). The finding of a variable effect on plasma androgen levels in the presence of a positive clinical response has been interpreted as indicating that the major effect of spironolactone is on the androgen receptor rather than on steroid production. Further support for this concept was obtained by Lobo et al (1985) who found that a similar decrease in plasma testosterone levels occurred in patients treated with 100 mg or 200 mg spironolactone. It is of interest that these authors also measured levels of DHT and Adiol-G. Whenever plasma DHT levels decreased during therapy, Adiol-G levels increased, raising further doubts about the usefulness of this androgen conjugate as a marker of peripheral androgen metabolism.

As spironolactone lacks the strong progestational action of CPA, two studies have examined the effect of combining spironolactone with oral contraceptive therapy. The combination of spironolactone with Conova (30 μg ethynyloestradiol plus 2 mg ethynodiol diacetate) produced an improvement in hirsutism as assessed by the Ferriman–Gallwey score (Chapman et al, 1985). Addition of the o.c. was thought to increase therapeutic effectiveness by decreasing gonadotrophin-mediated androgen secretion and also by increasing serum SHBG levels. Pittaway et al (1985) examined the effect of combining spironolactone with o.c. or dexamethasone therapy in women who had failed to show a clinical response to single drug therapy with o.c. or dexamethasone. The majority of patients showed an improvement in hair growth when treated with spironolactone combined with either o.c. or dexamethasone.

Several reports have commented upon the side-effects associated with the use of spironolactone. Shapiro and Evron (1980) found that 27% of women treated with 200 mg spironolactone developed menorrhagia and the development of menstrual irregularities in some treated patients was noted by Biffighandi et al (1984). Helfer et al (1988) compared the side-effects associated with the use of 200 mg and 100 mg spironolactone. In patients receiving 200 mg spironolactone the side-effects were severe enough to necessitate a reduction or discontinuation of the dose. For patients receiving 100 mg spironolactone only 2 of 10 women developed menorrhagia. Although this may not be considered to be a serious side-effect, women were reported to find it disturbing.

### CPA versus spironolactone

There have been few clearly designed trials to compare the use of CPA and spironolactone for the treatment of hirsutism. Lunde and Djoseland (1987) compared the effectiveness of 2 mg CPA plus ethinyloestradiol (50 µg) and spironolactone (50 mg). Marked differences in the effects of these two forms of therapy were observed. The dose of spironolactone examined did not affect plasma androgen levels, yet the reduction in hair growth was similar to that reported in response to higher doses. In contrast plasma androgen and gonadotrophin decreased in patients treated with CPA. While there was a significant improvement in the hair score parameters for patients treated with CPA, they were less marked than for patients treated with spirono-lactone. However, as noted by Lunde and Djoseland, the dose of CPA used is much less than that required to obtain a maximum clinical response.

### Topical administration of anti-androgens

Although there is a need for an anti-androgen that is effective after local application, no such compound has yet reached the stage of clinical trials. Bingham et al (1979) reported a decrease in sebaceous function after topical application of CPA in ethanol. However, this finding was not confirmed by Lyons and Shuster (1983) who applied CPA to the skin using ethanol or isopropyl myristate as a vehicle.

## MANAGEMENT OF ANTI-ANDROGEN THERAPY

### Indications for treatment and selection of patients

For women with mild hirsutism or well localized hair growth, simple cosmetic measures such as plucking, shaving, bleaching or electrolysis may provide a satisfactory means of controlling unwanted hair. Such methods, however, may produce insufficient improvement or may be distasteful to the patient and there is no reason why women with mild hirsutism should not be considered for anti-androgen treatment. In patients with moderate or severe hirsutism medical treatment is the most effective method of controlling the excessive hair growth. Severe or persistent acne and androgen-dependent alopecia are other clear indications for anti-androgen treatment (Miller and Jacobs, 1986).

The extent of the investigations prior to considering treatment partly depends on the interest of the centre to which the patient presents as well as the clinical context. But, as stated previously, it is clearly very important, in women with severe symptoms, to exclude more serious causes of hirsutism, such as virilizing tumour of the ovary or adrenal. Measurement of serum testosterone is in our experience a simple and useful screening procedure. If the concentration of testosterone exceeds 5.0 nmol/l (i.e. approximately twice the upper limit of the normal range in our assay) we undertake more extensive tests of ovarian and adrenal function.

As with the combined o.c., contraindications to treatment with CPA and ethinyloestradiol include a history of thromboembolic disease, hypertension and cigarette smoking.

### Choice and dose of anti-androgen

The data presented in this review point to the efficacy of CPA in controlling excessive body hair and acne. The results of treatment with spironolactone are less conclusive. Furthermore there is concern about possible toxicity of long-term usage of spironolactone which has prompted the Committee on Safety of Medicines to recommend that its use in the UK should be restricted to life-threatening conditions such as nephrotic syndrome and hepatic disease. For these reasons we use cyproterone as the treatment of choice. However, we recognize that CPA is not generally available in the USA.

The standard therapeutic regimen is, as outlined earlier in this review, a combination of CPA 100 mg daily from days 5–14 of cycle and ethinyl-oestradiol 50 µg/day for days 5–25. We find that the majority of patients experience a significant and satisfactory improvement if cyproterone is given at a starting dose of 50 mg daily. If this fails to achieve a significant reduction of hair growth after 6 months of treatment the dosage can be increased to 100 mg/day. The incidence of progestational side-effects such as breast tenderness and weight gain is lower on the smaller dose. It rarely seems necessary to use as much as 50 µg ethinyloestradiol. Ethinyloestradiol 30 µg/day between days 5 and 25 of the cycle with CPA 50 or 100 mg can be expected to provide good cycle control, without breakthrough bleeding and without loss of efficacy with regard either to suppression of hair growth or to contraception.

### Assessment of response to treatment

Subjective and clinical assessment by physician and patient is the most practical and, arguably, the most important means of assessing the response to anti-androgen therapy. Using the Ferrimen–Gallwey chart to measure the degree of hirsutism is a simple, semi-objective method and it is doubtful whether the more sophisticated methods such as photographic analysis or hair-weighing have any place in the setting of a routine clinic. These methods are more suited to research programmes where a quantitative assessment of change in hair growth is clearly important. Serum testosterone concentrations should fall during treatment and measurement of testosterone after 3 months' treatment will aid in the identification of patients with hypersecretion of adrenal androgens who would be expected to respond less well to CPA.

It is worth pointing out that in some patients acne may become transiently worse in the first few weeks of anti-androgen treatment but that the long-term results are usually extremely good.

## Duration of treatment and further medical management

As stated previously, most patients can be expected to experience a return of unwanted hair growth on stopping treatment with cyproterone. Long-term management is therefore difficult. Although there is little direct evidence that long-term treatment with high-dose cyproterone carries more risks than pro-longed use of conventional low-dose combined o.c., CPA is a progestogen with effects—albeit slight—on carbohydrate and lipid metabolism, and it would seem sensible to consider the use of lower doses of progestogen as soon as possible. Our approach is to continue treatment with high-dose cyproterone until the maximum improvement has been obtained (in practice this may take up to 12 months) and sustained for at least a further 12 months. Thus patients receive standard doses of CPA and ethinyloestradiol for 18–24 months. An alternative approach is to begin to reduce the dose of CPA as soon as maximum clinical improvement has been obtained, e.g. from 100 to 50 to 25 mg at 6-monthly intervals. Thereafter the improvement can be maintained in many patients by switching to a low-dose combined o.c. which contains a non-androgenic progestogen, i.e. avoiding the use of 19-norgestogens such as norgestrel (USP) or norethisterone which themselves have androgenic properties. The use of low-dose (2 mg) cyproterone has been advocated (see above), and with the recent availability of a combined pill containing only 35 µg ethinyloestradiol this seems an attractive choice. However, it remains to be determined whether cyproterone in this low dose has any advantage over any other non-androgenic progestogens such as desogestrel. Clearly, if changing to a low-dose contraceptive preparation fails to keep the hirsutism under control, there remains the option of continued treatment with high-dose cyproterone.

## SUMMARY

Hirsutism and acne in women are common distressing problems. Unwanted hair growth, acne and seborrhoea result from the action of androgens on the skin. Such effects depend not only on increased androgen production by the ovary or adrenal gland but also on the bioavailability of androgen to peripheral tissues. This in turn is related to transport of androgens in plasma by specific binding proteins and to peripheral metabolism of testosterone and androstenedione to their more potent 5α-reduced derivatives. An effective anti-androgen is one which blocks the androgen receptor-mediated actions of testosterone and DHT on skin. CPA, the treatment of choice in the UK, is a potent androgen receptor-blocking steroid which also has progestational properties. When combined with ethinyloestradiol it also suppresses ovarian function, thus reducing androgen production, and provides effective contraception.

# REFERENCES

Anderson DC (1974) Sex hormone binding globulin. *Clinical Endocrinology* **3:** 69–73.

Anderson KM & Liao S (1968) Selective retention of dihydrotestosterone by prostatic nuclei. *Nature* **219:** 277–279.

Barnes EW, Irvine WJ, Hunter WN & Ismail AAA (1975) Cyproterone acetate: a study involving two volunteers with idiopathic hirsutism. *Clinical Endocrinology* **4:** 65–73.

Baxendale PM, Jacobs HS & James VHT (1982) Salivary testosterone in normal and hyperandrogenic women. *Clinical Endocrinology* **16:** 595–603.

Baxendale PM, Jacobs HS & James VHT (1983) Plasma and salivary androstenedione and dihydrotestosterone in women with hyperandrogenism. *Clinical Endocrinology* **18:** 447–457.

Belisle S & Love EJ (1986) Clinical efficacy and safety of cyproterone acetate in severe hirsutism: results of a multicentered Canadian study. *Fertility and Sterility* **46:** 1015–1020.

Biffighandi P, Massacchetti C & Molinatti GM (1984) Female hirsutism: pathophysiological considerations and therapeutic implications. *Endocrine Reviews* **5:** 498–513.

Bingham KD, Low M & Wyatt EH (1979) Effect of topical cyproterone acetate on the sebum excretion in man. *Lancet* **ii:** 394–405.

Boisselle A & Tremblay RR (1979) New therapeutic approach to the hirsute patient. *Fertility and Sterility* **32:** 276–279.

Boisselle A, Dionne FT & Tremblay RR (1979) Interaction of spironolactone with rat skin androgen receptor. *Canadian Journal of Biochemistry* **57:** 1042–1046.

Bruchovsky N & Wilson JD (1968) Conversion of testosterone to 5α-androst-17β-ol-3-one by rat prostate in vivo and in vitro. *Journal of Biological Chemistry* **243:** 2012–2021.

Chapman MG, Jeffcoate SL & Dewhurst CJ (1982) Effect of cyproterone acetate–ethinyloestradiol treatment on adrenal function in hirsute women. *Clinical Endocrinology* **17:** 577–582.

Chapman MG, Dowsett M & Dewhurst CJ (1985) Spironolactone in combination with an oral contraceptive: an alternative treatment for hirsutism. *British Journal of Obstetrics and Gynaecology* **92:** 983–985.

Cheng RW, Reed MJ & James VHT (1986) Plasma free testosterone: equilibrium dialysis vs direct radioimmunoassay. *Clinical Chemistry* **32:** 1411.

Dorfman RI (1970) Biological activity of antiandrogens. *British Journal of Dermatology* **82:** 3–7.

Dunn JF, Nisula BC & Rodbard D (1981) Transport of steroid hormones: binding of 21 endogenous steroids to both testosterone-binding globulin and corticosteroid-binding globulin in human plasma. *Journal of Clinical Endocrinology and Metabolism* **53:** 58–68.

Evans DJ & Burke CW (1986) Spironolactone in the treatment of idiopathic hirsutism and the polycystic ovary syndrome. *Journal of the Royal Society of Medicine* **79:** 451–453.

Franks S, Adams J, Mason H & Polson D (1985) Ovulatory disorders in women with polycystic ovary syndrome. *Clinics in Obstetrics and Gynaecology* **12:** 605–632.

Frohlich M, Lachinsky N & Moolenaar AJ (1977) The influence of combined cyproterone acetate–ethinyloestradiol therapy on serum levels of dehydroepiandrosterone, androstenedione and testosterone in hirsute women. *Acta Endocrinologica (Copenhagen)* **84:** 333–342.

Giorgi EP (1980) The transport of steroid hormones into animal cells. *International Review of Cytology* **65:** 49–115.

Girard J, Baumann JB, Buhler U et al (1978) Cyproterone acetate and ACTH adrenal function. *Journal of Clinical Endocrinology and Metabolism* **47:** 581–586.

Giusti M, Parazzi F, Reitano A et al (1977) Longitudinal study of the behaviour of certain hormonal parameters in women undergoing treatment with cyproterone acetate. *Acta Europeaa Fertilitates* **8:** 211–228.

Goldzieher JW, Pena A & Aivaliotis MM (1978) Radio-immunoassay of androstenedione, testosterone and 11β-hydroxyandrostenedione after chromatography on Lipidex 5000. *Journal of Steroid Biochemistry* **9:** 169–173.

Hague WM, Munro DS, Sawers RS et al (1982) Long-term effects of cyproterone acetate on the pituitary adrenal axis in adult women. *British Journal of Obstetrics and Gynaecology* **89:** 981–984.

Hammerstein J & Cupceancu B (1969) Behandlung des Hirsutismus mit Cyproteronacetat. *Deutsche Medizinische Wochenschrift* **94:** 829–834.

Hammerstein J, Meckies J, Leo-Rossberg I et al (1975) Use of cyproterone acetate in the treatment of acne, hirsutism and virilism. *Journal of Steroid Biochemistry* **6:** 827–836.

Hammerstein J, Moltz L & Schwartz U (1983) Antiandrogens in the treatment of hirsutism. *Journal of Steroid Biochemistry* **19:** 591–597.

Helfer EL, Miller JL & Rose LI (1988) Side-effects of spironolactone therapy in the hirsute woman. *Journal of Clinical Endocrinology and Metabolism* **66:** 208–211.

Holdaway IM, Croxson MS, Evans MC et al (1983) Effect of cyproterone acetate on glucocorticoid secretion in patients treated for hirsutism. *Acta Endocrinologica* **104:** 222–226.

Holdaway IM, Croxson MS, Ibbertson HK et al (1985) Cyproterone acetate as initial treatment and maintenance therapy for hirsutism. *Acta Endocrinologica (Copenhagen)* **109:** 522–529.

Horton R & Lobo RA (eds) (1987) Androgen metabolism in hirsute and normal females. *Clinics in Endocrinology and Metabolism* **15:** 213–409.

Horton R, Lobo R & Hawks D (1982) Androstanediol glucuronide in plasma: a marker of androgen action. *Journal of Clinical Investigation* **69:** 1203–1206.

Ismail AAA, Davidson DW, Souka AR et al (1974) The evaluation of the role of androgens in hirsutism and the use of a new antiandrogen cyproterone acetate for therapy. *Journal of Clinical Endocrinology and Metabolism* **39:** 81–95.

Jeffcoate SL (ed.) (1982) *Androgens and Anti-androgen Therapy.* Chichester: John Wiley.

Jones EL & Woodbury L (1964) The effect of antiandrogens on the response of rat preputial glands to testosterone. *Journal of Investigative Dermatology* **43:** 165–169.

Kirschner MA & Jacobs J (1971) Combined ovarian and adrenal vein catheterization to determine the sites of androgen production in hirsute women. *Journal of Clinical Endocrinology and Metabolism* **33:** 199–209.

Kirschner MA, Zucker IR & Jespersen DL (1976) Ovarian and adrenal vein catheterization studies in women with idiopathic hirsutism. In James VHT, Serio M & Giusti G (eds) *The Endocrine Function of the Human Ovary*, pp 443–456. London: Academic Press.

Lobo RA, Shoupe D, Serafini P et al (1985) The effects of two doses of spironolactone on serum androgens and androgen hair in hirsute women. *Fertility and Sterility* **43:** 200–205.

Lunde O & Djoseland O (1987) A comparative study of Aldactone and Diane in the treatment of hirsutism. *Journal of Steroid Biochemistry* **28:** 161–165.

Lunnell NO, Zador G, Carlstrom K et al (1982) The effect of cyproterone acetate on pituitary ovarian function and clinical symptoms in hirsute women. *Acta Endocrinologica (Copenhagen)* **100:** 91–97.

Lyons F & Shuster S (1983) Indirect evidence that the action of cyproterone acetate on the skin is due to a metabolite. *Clinical Endocrinology* **19:** 53–55.

Menhard RH, Bartter FC & Gillette JR (1976) Spironolactone and cytochrome P-450: impairment of steroid 21-hydroxylation in the adrenal cortex. *Archives of Biochemistry and Biophysics* **173:** 395.

Milewicz A, Silber D & Kirschner MA (1983) Therapeutic effects of spironolactone in polycystic ovary syndrome. *Obstetrics and Gynecology* **61:** 429–432.

Miller JA, Jacobs HS (1986) Treatment of hirsutism and acne with cyproterone acetate. *Clinics in Endocrinology and Metabolism* **15:** 373–389.

Mowszowicz I, Melanitou E, Kirchhoffer MO & Mauvais-Jarvis P (1983) Dihydrotestosterone stimulates 5α-reductase activity in pubic skin fibroblasts. *Journal of Clinical Endocrinology and Metabolism* **56:** 320–325.

Pardridge WM & Mietus LJ (1979) Transport of steroid hormones through the blood–brain barrier. Primary role of albumin-bound hormone. *Journal of Clinical Investigation* **64:** 745–752.

Pittaway DE, Maxson WS & Wentz AC (1985) Spironolactone in combination drug therapy for unresponsive hirsutism. *Fertility and Sterility* **43:** 878–882.

Polson DW, Reed MJ, Franks S et al (1988) Serum 11β-hydroxyandrostenedione as an indicator of the source of excess androgen production in women with polycystic ovaries. *Journal of Clinical Endocrinology and Metabolism* **66:** 946–950.

Poran J, Guber A, Schindler D & Shachor Y (1986) Pulmonary embolism after short-term treatment of acne vulgaris with ovulation suppressor agents. *Medical Journal of Australia* **145:** 345.

Reed MJ, Whorwood CB, Scanlon MJ et al (1986) Regulation of plasma levels of 3α-androstanediol glucuronide. In Genazzani AR, Volpe A & Facchinetti F (eds) *Research on Gynaecological Endocrinology*, pp 199–202. Carnforth: Parthenon Publishing.

Rose LI, Underwood RH, Newmark SR et al (1977) Pathophysiology of spironolactone induced gynaecomastia. *Annals of Internal Medicine* **87:** 397–403.

Rubens R (1984) Androgen levels during cyproterone acetate and ethinyloestradiol treatment of hirsutism. *Clinical Endocrinology* **20:** 313–325.

Scanlon MJ, Whorwood CB, Reed MJ et al (1987) Androsterone glucuronide—a marker of peripheral androgen metabolism. *Journal of Endocrinology* **115 (suppl):** abstract 131.

Scanlon MJ, Whorwood CB, Franks S et al (1988) Serum androstanediol glucuronide concentrations in normal and hirsute women and patients with thyroid dysfunction. *Clinical Endocrinology* (in press).

Seed M, Godsland IF, Wynn V & Jacobs HS (1984) The effects of cyproterone acetate and ethinyloestradiol on carbohydrate metabolism. *Clinical Endocrinology* **21:** 689–699.

Shapiro G & Evron S (1980) A novel use of spironolactone: treatment of hirsutism. *Journal of Clinical Endocrinology and Metabolism* **51:** 429–432.

Siiteri PK, Murai JT, Hammond GL, Nisker JA, Raymoure WJ & Kuhn RW (1982) The serum transport of steroid hormones. *Recent Progress in Hormone Research* **38:** 457–510.

Stahl ML, Teeslink CR & Greenblatt RD (1973) Ovarian, adrenal and peripheral testosterone levels in the polycystic ovary syndrome. *American Journal of Obstetrics and Gynecology* **117:** 194–200.

Stivel MS, Kauli R, Kaufman H & Laron Z (1982) Adrenocortical function in children with precocious sexual development during treatment with cyproterone acetate. *Clinical Endocrinology* **16:** 163–169.

Underhill R & Dewhurst J (1979) Further clinical experience in the treatment of hirsutism with cyproterone acetate. *British Journal of Obstetrics and Gynaecology* **86:** 139–141.

Vermeulen A (1979) The androgens. In Gray CH & James VHT (eds) *Hormones in Blood*, vol. 3, pp 355–416. London: Academic Press.

Wynn V, Godsland IF, Seed M et al (1986) Paradoxical effects of the anti-androgen cyproterone acetate on lipid and lipoprotein metabolism. *Clinical Endocrinology* **24:** 183–191.

Young RL, Goldzieher JW & Elkind-Hirsch K (1987) The endocrine effects of spironolactone as an antiandrogen. *Fertility and Sterility* **48:** 223–228.

Zielske F, Leo-Rossberg I, Dreykluft RM et al (1971) Treatment of hirsutism and signs of virilism with a reversed sequential administration of cyproterone acetate and ethinyl-oestradiol. Clinical and endocrinological aspects. *Acta Endocrinologica (Copenhagen)* **suppl. 155:** 172.

# 5

# Anti-progesterones: background and clinical physiology

I. T. CAMERON
D. L. HEALY

## ANTI-PROGESTERONE AGENTS: RATIONALE AND DEVELOPMENT

The potential clinical impact of anti-progesterone agents can be more clearly appreciated after considering the physiological roles of both progesterone and its receptor. Few physiological studies have been undertaken of progesterone action in the human uterus. Indeed, the progesterone receptor was characterized initially for the chick oviduct. The receptor in both the chick and human is a protein dimer with subunits A and B of 80 000 and 110 000 daltons respectively. Both subunits bind progesterone and DNA (Horwitz et al, 1985).

Direct analysis of the structure of the progesterone receptor has been hampered because of the low concentrations and lability of these important regulatory proteins. Molecular cloning advances have recently allowed the determination of the amino acid sequences of the glucocorticoid and oestrogen receptors. More recently, the cloning of the progesterone receptor genes from the rabbit and from the chick oviduct have been reported (Loosfelt et al, 1986; Conneely et al, 1986). The comparison of rabbit and human progesterone receptors did indicate regions of the amino acid sequence that were highly conserved and therefore may have similar biological functions. For this reason, a cDNA probe encoding the rabbit progesterone receptor has been recently used to screen a library containing DNAs complementary to messenger RNAs from a human breast cancer cell line (T47-D) in order to derive the complete amino acid sequence of the human progesterone receptor (Misrahi et al, 1987). This work indicates that the human progesterone receptor is a protein of 933 amino acids with a molecular weight of 98 868 daltons. The protein contains a cysteine basic region which appears to be involved in DNA binding and is completely homologous between the human and rabbit progesterone receptors. The C-terminal end, where binding with progesterone is thought to take place, differs by only a single amino acid change and the human progesterone receptor is characterized by a very high content of the amino acid proline at its N-terminal region. The availability of molecular probes of this type for the human progesterone receptor should now permit the analysis of the expression of this gene throughout the human genital tract.

Progesterone binds to the complete receptor with a high affinity, but the resultant complex dissociates rapidly. The steroid also binds with similar affinity to transcortin or corticosteroid-binding globulin (CBG). This is clinically relevant, for the concentration of CBG in endometrium usually exceeds that of the conventional progesterone receptor. Other steroids, oestradiol, cortisol and testosterone, have negligible affinity for the progesterone receptor.

The progesterone receptor is one of several proteins synthesized by the action of oestradiol on the endometrial epithelial and stromal cells in the proliferative phase of the menstrual cycle. Indeed, progesterone receptors appear in these cells early in the proliferative phase, several days before progesterone secretion by the corpus luteum. Approximately 12 000 progesterone receptors per endometrial cell are present at mid-cycle when their concentration is approximately 3.0 pmol/mg DNA. As progesterone is increasingly secreted by the corpus luteum after ovulation, the total number of progesterone receptors falls progressively in the endometrial cells throughout the luteal phase. This appears to be due to 'down-regulation' of the steroid upon its own receptor (Walters and Clark, 1979).

Until recently, a major tenet of steroid hormone dogma was that there were cytoplasmic steroid receptors which could translocate into the nucleus after binding to the particular steroid to result in the synthesis, or inhibition of synthesis, of specific proteins. Two major studies have recently suggested that this concept is wrong and that steroid receptors, such as those for progesterone or oestradiol, are located only in the nucleus of the endometrial cell (King and Greene, 1984; Welshons et al, 1984).

However it arrives in the nucleus, progesterone has several actions through the genome of both endometrial glandular and stromal cells. It increases endometrial inactivation of oestradiol 17-dehydrogenase in glandular epithelium; this mechanism decreases the ratio of nuclear oestradiol to oestrone and thereby decreases endometrial DNA synthesis (Tseng and Gurpide, 1975). The progesterone receptor also allows synthesis of several endometrial proteins. These include prolactin, which is secreted by endometrial stromal cells and the progestagen-associated endometrial protein (PEP; α-uteroprotein) which is secreted by endometrial epithelial cells, as well as inhibitors of plasminogen activator (Healy and Hodgen, 1983). Furthermore, progesterone appears to play an important role in the storage and regulation of endometrial prostaglandin production (Smith et al, 1982; Cameron et al, 1987).

Progesterone receptor physiology during pregnancy is even less well understood. In non-human primates, progesterone acts through its endometrial receptor in early pregnancy to increase fivefold the ratio of endometrial oestrone to oestradiol binding (Kreitmann-Gimbal et al, 1981). It is widely accepted that progesterone helps to prevent premature human labour by blocking myometrial contractility by increasing calcium binding to the sarcoplasmic reticulum and myometrial cell membrane (Csapo, 1977). Nevertheless, unlike the sheep, human labour has never been shown to follow a sudden fall in progesterone production. In two prospective series of normal term primigravid patients, only some women showed decreases in plasma progesterone levels prior to labour and these decreases were gradual rather than acute (Csapo et al, 1971; Turnbull et al, 1974). In the latter study, mean plasma progesterone concentrations were 169 ng/ml at 36 weeks gestation and 103 ng/ml in labour. Progesterone levels 1 week before labour were equivalent to those measured during labour. No study has yet examined primate periplacental or amniochorionic progesterone concentrations, or its receptor physiology before or during birth. It is surely here, and not in peripheral blood, that progesterone exerts its physiological role.

In the light of these actions of progesterone, the possible clinical applications of agents that would inhibit the steroid have become apparent. For some time therefore, attempts have been made to develop anti-progesterone agents with relatively few side-effects. Earlier compounds included gestrinone (R-2323), anordrin and ORF 9371 (Sakiz et al, 1974; Mora et al, 1975; Gu and Chang, 1979; Hahn et al, 1980). However the therapeutic potential of many of these agents was limited, either because of androgenic side-effects, or as a result of inadequate clinical efficacy.

An alternative approach was to inhibit ovarian progesterone synthesis. This is more difficult than it sounds because any administered drug will also inhibit the biosynthesis of progesterone and related steroids in the adrenal gland. Nevertheless, inhibitors of the enzyme 3β-hydroxysteroid dehydrogenase such as trilostane or epostane have been reported consistently to impair progesterone synthesis in human beings (Van Der Spuy et al, 1983; Webster et al, 1985).

## CLINICAL PHARMACOLOGY OF PROGESTERONE RECEPTOR ANTAGONISTS

Biochemical analysis of the steroid structure of progesterone indicates that it is a planar molecule. By contrast, the norethindrone-derived anti-progesterones mifepristone (RU 486; Roussel-Uclaf, Paris) and ZK98734 (Schering AG, Berlin) possess a hydrophobic moiety at position 11, a configuration which appears essential for progesterone receptor-blocking actions (Figure 1).

Many synthetic variations of these structures are possible (Teutsch, 1981; Neef et al, 1984). It appears very difficult to dissociate the affinity of these compounds for the progesterone receptor on the one hand and for the glucocorticoid receptor on the other. Currently there is no pure progester-

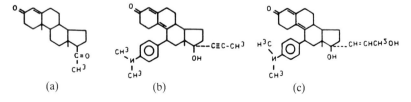

**Figure 1.** The structures of (a) progesterone, (b) mifepristone and (c) ZK98734.

one antagonist or pure glucocorticoid antagonist which is sufficiently active in vivo to be clinically useful, though following mifepristone administration to women, no impairment of the hypothalamo-pituitary-adrenal axis has been seen using doses that stimulate uterine contractility (Gaillard et al, 1984).

In vitro pharmacological studies have been best characterized with the anti-progesterone mifepristone. This compound binds to the progesterone receptor five times more avidly than does progesterone in the uterus of the female rabbit pretreated with oestradiol. It also binds to the glucocorticoid receptor of the adrenalectomized rat thymus three times more strongly than dexamethasone. By contrast, it binds to the androgen receptor of the castrated rat prostate with only one-quarter of the affinity of testosterone and has essentially no binding to the mineralocorticoid receptor of the adrenalectomized rat kidney or the oestrogen receptor of the immature mouse (Philibert et al, 1981).

In vivo, at an oral dose of 3–30 mg/kg, mifepristone inhibited the action of exogenous progesterone on the endometrium of the immature rabbit pre-treated with oestradiol. It also inhibited both deciduoma formation induced by 150 mg progesterone and the occurrence of giant mitochondria induced by 20 mg progesterone subcutaneously. In none of the above tests did mifepristone manifest any progestomimetic activity (see below).

The bioavailability of mifepristone in man appears to be 30–56% of the administered dose, with 85% of the steroid being absorbed after oral therapy. Mifepristone binds strongly to α-1 acid glycoprotein and to a lesser extent to albumin. This results in a long half-life—about 12 hours following intravenous administration, and 24 hours orally—leading to a slow metabolic clearance (Deraedt, 1984). The major metabolite of mifepristone, the N-demethylated RU42633, also possesses anti-progesterone and anti-glucocorticoid activity, albeit with a much reduced potency than its parent compound.

No acute toxic effects have been seen in the mouse following administration of mifepristone at doses of 800–1000 mg/kg intraperitoneally or orally. A 30-day toxicity test in rats given up to 200 mg/kg orally showed no mortality, but retarded growth and endometrial and adrenal changes consistent with the hormonal activities of the compound were observed. A 30-day toxicity test in monkeys at 100 mg/kg orally resulted in weight loss, decreased appetite and diarrhoea. The expected changes in adrenal function consistent with an anti-glucocorticoid action were observed.

Embryotoxicity is difficult to evaluate in a compound whose major mode of action is likely to be pregnancy interruption. No teratogenic effects have been seen in the rat or rabbit with mifepristone at doses of 1 mg/kg, and no mutagenic action was observed on bacteriological testing (Healy, 1985).

## PHYSIOLOGICAL STUDIES

### Non-human primate

A number of studies have now been reported using the macaque monkey as a model for the potential endocrine effects of mifepristone in humans. Initial studies investigated whether menstrual induction with mifepristone was the result of a direct endometrial action, or a consequence of luteolysis.

Adult female cynomologus monkeys (*Macaca fascicularis*) were castrated at least 2 months prior to experimentation. Each animal received a schedule of silastic capsules over a 49-day course. These capsules contained oestradiol or progesterone and were administered in a regimen previously shown to mimic the circulating steroidal milieu of the normal ovarian cycle and early pregnancy in monkeys (Healy et al, 1983). Each animal received vehicle only or mifepristone on days 31–34 of each 49-day treatment cycle.

Menses occurred in all primates injected with fully solubilized mifepristone, regardless of the dose of the drug given (0.1–10 mg/kg). Bleeding began within 72 hours of the first injection in 9 animals, and persisted for at least 3 days in 8 cases. Menstruation did not occur following the injection of vehicle alone. Furthermore, all monkeys which menstruated during or after mifepristone administration also bled within 72 hours of removal of the exogenous oestradiol and progesterone capsules at the end of the treatment cycle. Mifepristone could therefore induce menses by a direct action on the endometrium, and later studies confirmed this finding in intact monkeys in both the pregnant and non-pregnant states (Healy and Hodgen, 1985).

Further work examined the morphological response to administration of the anti-progestin. A marked thinning of the endometrium occurred within 18 hours of mifepristone exposure, and after 32 hours haemorrhagic lakes were seen in the superficial zone, with desquamation of the epithelium within the lumina of the endometrial glands. Menstruation was observed after at least 44 hours (Koering et al, 1985).

The monkey has also been used to examine the effects of mifepristone on the hypothalamo-pituitary-adrenal axis. Castrated cynomologus monkeys were given 30 days of steroid replacement with oestradiol and progesterone. Following the injection of mifepristone (10 mg/kg), blood samples were taken at frequent intervals for up to 8 hours via chronically indwelling cannulae (Sopelak et al, 1983).

Plasma levels of adrenocorticotrophin (ACTH), arginine vasopressin (AVP) and cortisol increased after mifepristone treatment, and more recent data have confirmed a dose-related relationship with the anti-glucocorticoid activity (Healy et al, 1985). This work also revealed a 50-fold difference (0.1 versus 5.0 mg/kg) between a significant endometrial response and a significant anti-glucocorticoid action, in keeping with previous studies (Gaillard et al, 1984).

The administration of anti-progesterone steroids at different stages of the spontaneous menstrual cycle has also been assessed (Collins et al, 1985). Three of four monkeys showed a significant reduction in luteinizing hormone (LH) pulse frequency and amplitude following mifepristone treatment on day 13 of the ovarian cycle, suggesting that anti-progesterones may block the synergistic action of progesterone in the oestradiol-induced pre-ovulatory LH surge. Further studies confirmed the ability of mifepristone to inhibit the mid-cycle LH surge, resulting in loss of the dominant follicle and the anticipated 2-week delay to ovulation and subsequent menstruation (Collins and Hodgen, 1966).

## Human

The first clinical trials of mifepristone, administered at a dose of 200 mg/day for 4 days to women between 6 and 8 weeks pregnant produced abortion in 9 of 11 individuals. Treatment in the mid-luteal phase led to menstruation within 2 days (Herrmann et al, 1982). These effects were ascribed to progesterone receptor antagonistic activity at the target tissue. Subsequent physiological studies have suggested that the anti-progestins may act not only directly at the level of the endometrium, but also by reducing pituitary gonadotrophin release, or by inhibiting ovarian steroidogenesis (Figure 2).

The administration of mifepristone 25–100 mg/day from days 19–23 of the cycle induced bleeding within 4 days in 29 of 32 women (Schaison et al, 1985). In 15 cases a further bleed was seen at the expected time of menstru-

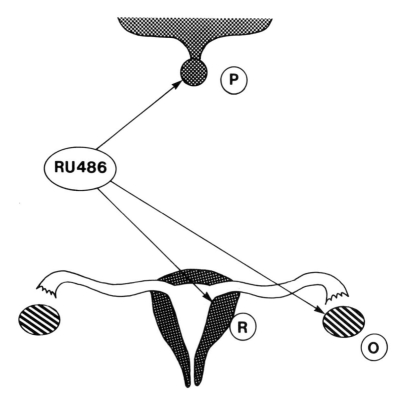

**Figure 2.** Mifepristone (RU486): sites of action. R = endometrial progesterone receptor (menses induction and increases in prostaglandin production); P = impaired pituitary gonadotrophin secretion; O = modified ovarian steroidogenesis (reduced 17-hydroxylase activity and progesterone production).

ation, implying that mifepristone had acted at the endometrial receptor level to induce bleeding in the absence of luteolysis. Circulating LH and follicle-stimulating hormone concentrations were measured in 17 women. Gonado-trophin inhibition was seen in 10 cases; however, luteal regression was only seen in 5 individuals, and in a further 2 cases, corpus luteum regression was seen in the absence of a change in LH concentrations. Circulating cortisol or ACTH levels were not affected in 7 women, receiving 100 mg mifepristone daily for 4 days, in whom these parameters were measured.

An inhibitory effect of mifepristone on pituitary gonadotrophin release was also reported in postmenopausal women (Gravanis et al, 1985). Pro-gesterone or mifepristone was given either alone or in combination to groups of 2 or 3 women who had already received 9 days of oestradiol priming. Oestradiol alone reduced postmenopausal gonadotrophin concen-trations, and a further suppression was seen with progesterone or mife-pristone, or progesterone plus mifepristone, confirming that mifepristone may have partial agonist activity, with its progestogenic activity being unmasked in the absence of endogenous progesterone. Similar partial agonist actions were also evident on assessing the endometrium histologi-cally and biochemically (DNA polymerase and oestradiol dehydrogenase activity).

As a consequence of their receptor-blocking actions, the anti-progester-one agents exert specific effects on progesterone-mediated events, such as endometrial prostaglandin production. Both mifepristone and ZK98734 stimulated prostaglandin production from endometrial stroma more than glands in short-term in vitro studies (Kelly et al, 1986). This work has recently been extended, revealing that the anti-progesterones stimulate the synthesis of prostaglandins $E_2$ and $F_{2\alpha}$ from glandular cells in early human decidua, but not stroma, and that the stimulation involves an effect on cyclo-oxygenase activity, and not an effect on the availability of precursor arachidonic acid (Smith and Kelly, 1987).

The observed action of mifepristone depends to a great extent on the timing of its administration. Given in the late luteal phase (days 23–27), at the normal time of endogenous progesterone withdrawal, mifepristone resulted in the consistent induction of bleeding after an interval of 1–3 days in 28 of 30 treatment cycles (Croxatto et al, 1987). Though the luteal phase of the treatment cycle was shortened by 1 or 2 days, the subsequent follicular phase was correspondingly longer, resulting in no overall disruption of the menstrual rhythm, but implying a dissociation between the 'clock' which times the LH surge, and that which signals the end of progesterone's action in the previous luteal phase. However, a delay to ovulation of 32 days was seen following luteal-phase menstrual induction with mifepristone in rhesus monkeys (Hodgen, 1985).

Different effects are seen when the anti-progesterones are administered to women with normal cycles in the follicular phase. Given on days 11–13, after the emergence of the dominant follicle, 3 mg/kg mifepristone for 3 days resulted in a reduction in oestradiol concentrations, followed by a rebound increase in gonadotrophin release leading to renewed folliculogenesis and the commencement of a new cycle. The mid-cycle LH surge was delayed by

15 days, and the fall in circulating oestradiol was associated with a decrease in the size, or a collapse, of the dominant follicle (Liu et al, 1987). There was no bleeding, and no change in LH pulse frequency or amplitude.

Besides these progesterone receptor-mediated actions, both centrally and at the level of the endometrium, mifepristone also appears to modify ovarian steroidogenesis (Figure 2). A dose-dependent suppression of progesterone production from cultured human granulosa cells has been reported (DiMattina et al, 1986), and subsequent studies have suggested an additional inhibitory effect on 17-hydroxylase activity (DiMattina et al, 1987).

## CLINICAL STUDIES

The main clinical application of the anti-progesterone steroids has been for the interruption of pregnancy, either for therapeutic abortion or for the induction of labour following fetal death in utero (Cabrol et al, 1985). Although effective at inducing menstruation in early pregnancy, by itself mifepristone is associated with an unacceptably high incidence of incomplete or unsuccessful abortion (Kovacs et al, 1984; Cameron et al, 1986; Couzinet et al, 1986). However, the addition of a subtherapeutic dose of prostaglandin following anti-progesterone priming has resulted in a success rate for medical abortion similar to that for vacuum aspiration (Swahn et al, 1985; Cameron and Baird, 1988).

## SUMMARY

The development of anti-progesterones has provided a probe to examine the role of progesterone both in the normal cycle and in pregnancy. The most widely used of these agents, mifepristone, appears to act both directly at the endometrial progesterone receptor, and centrally by reducing circulating gonadotrophin concentrations. In addition, ovarian steroidogenesis may be modified. The clinical application of these agents for the interruption of pregnancy will be considered in the following chapters.

## REFERENCES

Cabrol D, Bouvier D'Yvoire M, Mermet E, Cedard L, Sureau C & Baulieu EE (1985) Induction of labour with mifepristone after intra-uterine fetal death. *Lancet* ii: 1019.
Cameron IT & Baird DT (1988) Early pregnancy termination: a comparison between vacuum aspiration and medical abortion using prostaglandin (16, 16 dimethyl-trans-$\Delta_2$-PGE$_1$, methyl ester) or the anti-progestogen RU486. *British Journal of Obstetrics and Gynaecology* **95**: 271–276.
Cameron IT, Michie AF & Baird DT (1986) Therapeutic abortion in early pregnancy with anti-progestogen RU486 alone or in combination with prostaglandin analogue (gemeprost). *Contraception* **34**: 459–468.
Cameron IT, Leask R, Kelly RW & Baird DT (1987) The effects of danazol, mefenamic acid,

norethisterone, and a progesterone-impregnated coil, on endometrial prostaglandin concentrations in women with menorrhagia. *Prostaglandins* **34**: 99–110.

Collins RL & Hodgen GD (1986) Blockade of the spontaneous midcycle gonadotropin surge in monkeys by RU486: a progesterone antagonist or agonist? *Journal of Clinical Endocrinology and Metabolism* **63**: 1270–1276.

Collins RL, Healy DL & Hodgen GD (1985) Effects of RU486 on pulsatile gonadotropin secretion in monkeys throughout the ovarian menstrual cycle. *American Fertility Society Abstract* 72.

Conneely OM, Sullivan WP, Toft DO et al (1986) Molecular cloning of the chicken progesterone receptor. *Science* **233**: 767–770.

Couzinet B, Le Strat N, Ulmann A, Baulieu EE & Schaison G (1986) Termination of early pregnancy by progesterone antagonist RU486 (mifepristone). *New England Journal of Medicine* **315**: 1565–1570.

Croxatto HB, Salvatierra AM, Romero C & Spitz IM (1987) Late luteal phase administration of RU486 for three successive cycles does not disrupt bleeding patterns or ovulation. *Journal of Clinical Endocrinology and Metabolism* **65**: 1272–1277.

Csapo AL (1977) The see-saw theory of parturition. *Ciba Foundation Symposium* **47**: 159.

Csapo AL, Knobil E, Van Der Molen HJ & Weist WG (1971) Peripheral plasma progesterone levels during human pregnancy and labour. *American Journal of Obstetrics and Gynecology* **110**: 630–632.

Deraedt R (1984) The toxicology and pharmakokinetics of RU486. In Baulieu EE & Segal SJ (eds) *The antiprogestin steroid RU486 and human fertility control*, pp 155–163. New York: Plenum.

DiMattina M, Albertson B, Seyler DE, Loriaux DL & Falk RJ (1986) Effect of the antiprogestin RU486 on progesterone production by cultured human granulosa cells: inhibition of the ovarian 3β-hydroxysteroid dehydrogenase. *Contraception* **34**: 199–206.

DiMattina M, Albertson BD, Tyson V, Loriaux DL & Falk RJ (1987) Effect of the antiprogestin RU486 on human ovarian steroidogenesis. *Fertility and Sterility* **48**: 229–233.

Gaillard RC, Riondel A, Muller AF, Herrmann W & Baulieu EE (1984) RU486: a steroid with antiglucocorticosteroid activity that only disinhibits the pituitary adrenal system at a specific time of day. *Proceedings of the National Academy of Science, USA* **81**: 3879.

Gravanis A, Schaison G, George M et al (1985) Endometrial and pituitary responses to the steroidal antiprogestin RU486 in postmenopausal women. *Journal of Clinical Endocrinology and Metabolism* **60**: 156–163.

Gu Z & Chang MC (1979) A-nor steroids as post-coital contraceptives in the hampster with special reference to the transport and degeneration of eggs. *Contraception* **20**: 549–557.

Hahn BW, McGuire JL & Chang MC (1980) Contragestational agents. In Zatuchni GI, Labbok MH & Sciarra JJ (eds) *Research Frontiers in Fertility Regulation*, pp 246–261. Hagerstown: Harper & Row.

Healy DL (1985) Clinical status of antiprogesterone steroids. *Clinical Reproduction and Fertility* **3**: 277–296.

Healy DL & Hodgen GD (1983) The endocrinology of human endometrium. *Obstetrical and Gynecological Survey* **38**: 509–530.

Healy DL & Hodgen GD (1985) Non-human primate studies with RU486. In Baulieu EE & Segal SJ (eds) *The antiprogestin steroid RU486 and human fertility control*, pp 127–140. New York: Plenum.

Healy DL, Baulieu EE & Hodgen GD (1983) Induction of menstruation by an anti-progesterone steroid (RU486) in primates. Site of action, dose–response relationships and hormonal effects. *Fertility and Sterility* **40**: 253–257.

Healy DL, Chrousos GP, Schulte HM, Gold CW & Hodgen GD (1985) Increased adrenocorticotropin, cortisol and arginine vasopressin secretion in primates after the antiglucocorticoid steroid RU486: dose response relationships. *Journal of Clinical Endocrinology and Metabolism* **60**: 1.

Herrmann W, Wyss R, Riondel A et al (1982) The effects of an anti-progesterone steroid in women: interruption of the menstrual cycle and of early pregnancy. *Comptes Rendues* **294**: 933.

Hodgen GD (1985) Pregnancy prevention by intravaginal delivery of a progesterone antagonist: RU486 tampon for menstrual induction and absorption. *Fertility and Sterility* **44**: 263–267.

Horowitz KB, Wei LL, Sedlacek SM & D'Arville CN (1985) Progesterone action and progesterone receptor structure in human breast cancer: a review. *Recent Progress in Hormone Research* **41**: 249–316.

Kelly RW, Healy DL, Cameron MJ, Cameron IT & Baird DT (1986) The stimulation of prostaglandin production by two anti-progesterone steroids in human endometrial cells. *Journal of Clinical Endocrinology and Metabolism* **62**: 1116–1123.

King WJ & Greene GL (1984) Monoclonal antibodies localise oestrogen receptor in the nuclear target cells. *Nature* **307**: 745.

Koering MJ, Healy DL & Hodgen GD (1985) Morphological response of endometrium to progesterone antagonists in monkeys. *Fertility and Sterility* **45**: 280–287.

Kovacs L, Sas N, Resch RA et al (1984) Termination of very early pregnancy by RU486—an antiprogestational compound. *Contraception* **29**: 399–410.

Kreitmann-Gimbal B, Bayard F & Hodgen GD (1981) Changing ratios of nuclear oestrone to oestradiol binding in endometrium at implantation: regulation by chorionic gonadotropin and progesterone during rescue of the primate corpus luteum. *Journal of Clinical Endocrinology and Metabolism* **52**: 133–137.

Liu JH, Garzo G, Morris S, Stuenkel C, Ulmann A & Yen SCC (1987) Disruption of follicular maturation and delay of ovulation after administration of the antiprogesterone RU486. *Journal of Clinical Endocrinology and Metabolism* **65**: 1135–1140.

Loosfelt H, Atger M, Misrahi M et al (1986) Cloning and sequence analysis of rabbit progesterone receptor complementary DNA. *Proceedings of the National Academy of Science, USA* **83**: 9045–9049.

Misrahi M, Atger M, D'Auriol L et al (1987) The complete amino acid sequence of the human progesterone receptor deduced from clone to cDNA. *Biochemical and Biophysical Research Communications* **143**: 740–748.

Mora G, Faundes A & Johannson EBD (1975) Lack of clinical contraceptive efficacy of large doses of R-2323 given before implantation or after a missed period. *Contraception* **12**: 211–220.

Neef G, Sauer G, Seeger A & Wiechert R (1984) Synthetic variations of the progesterone antagonist RU38486. *Tetrahedron Letters* **25**: 3425.

Philibert D, Deraedt R & Teutsch G (1981) RU38486, a potent antiglucocorticoid in vivo. In *The 8th International Congress of Pharmacology*, Tokyo, Japan. Abstract 1463.

Sakiz E, Azadian-Boulanger G, Larague F & Raynaud JP (1974) A new approach to oestrogen-free contraception based on progesterone receptor blockade by mid-cycle administration of ethyl-norgestrienone (R-2323). *Contraception* **10**: 467–474.

Schaison G, George M, Lestrat N, Reinberg A & Baulieu EE (1985) Effects of the antiprogesterone steroid RU486 during midluteal phase in normal women. *Journal of Clinical Endocrinology and Metabolism* **61**: 484–489.

Smith SK & Kelly RW (1987) The effect of the antiprogestins RU486 and ZK98734 on the synthesis and metabolism of prostaglandins $F_{2\alpha}$ and $E_2$ in separated cells from early human decidua. *Journal of Clinical Endocrinology and Metabolism* **65**: 527–534.

Smith SK, Abel MH, Kelly RW & Baird DT (1982) The synthesis of prostaglandins from persistent proliferative endometrium. *Journal of Clinical Endocrinology and Metabolism* **55**: 284–289.

Sopelak VM, Lynch A, Williams RF & Hodgen GD (1983) Maintenance of ovulatory menstrual cycles in chronically cannulated monkeys: a vest and mobile tether assembly. *Biology of Reproduction* **28**: 703–706.

Swahn ML, Cekan S, Wong G, Lundstrom V, Bygdeman M (1985) Pharmakokinetic and clinical studies of RU486 for fertility regulation. In Baulieu EE & Segal SJ (eds), pp 249–258. *The Antiprogestin Steroid RU468 and Human Fertility Control*. New York: Plenum Press.

Teutsch G (1981) The chemistry of the antiprogesterone steroids. In Baulieu EE & Segal SJ (eds) *The antiprogestin steroid RU486 and human fertility control*, pp 178–190. New York: Plenum.

Tseng L & Gurpide E (1975) The effects of progestins on oestradiol receptor levels in human endometrium. *Journal of Clinical Endocrinology and Metabolism* **41**: 402–404.

Turnbull AC, Patten PY, Flint APE, Keirse MJNC, Jeremy JY & Anderson ABM (1974) Significant fall in progesterone and rise in oestradiol levels in human peripheral plasma before the onset of labour. *Lancet* **i**: 101–104.

Van Der Spuy SM, Jones DL, Wright CSW et al (1983) Inhibition of 3-beta-hydroxysteroid dehydrogenase activity in first trimester human pregnancy with trilostane and WIN32729. *Clinical Endocrinology* **19**: 521.

Walters MR & Clark JH (1979) Relationship between the quantity of progesterone receptor and the antagonism of oestrogen-induced uterotropic response. *Endocrinology* **105**: 382.

Webster MA, Phipps SL & Gilmer MDG (1985) Interruption of first trimester human pregnancy following epostane therapy. Effect of prostaglandin $E_2$ pessaries. *British Journal of Obstetrics and Gynaecology* **92**: 963–968.

Welshons WV, Lieberman ME & Gorski J (1984) Nuclear localization of unoccupied oestrogen receptors. *Nature* **307**: 747.

# 6

The use of anti-progesterones as a medical IUD

LYNNETTE K. NIEMAN
D. LYNN LORIAUX

Progesterone is essential for normal reproductive function in women. It governs the transformation of the endometrium from a proliferative to a secretory state and enables the nidation of a fertilized egg. Continued progesterone production by the corpus luteum is necessary for the process of placentation and for maintenance of early pregnancy. If progesterone secretion is subnormal, the endometrium does not develop normally and implantation cannot occur or is not sustained. This situation, called corpus luteum deficiency, is manifest as infertility or repeated miscarriages. The importance of progesterone to the integrity of the endometrium is illustrated in non-pregnant cycles by the timing of menses, which occur when progesterone levels decrease.

A progesterone antagonist could, in theory, interrupt the support of endogenous progesterone on the endometrium and prevent nidation. This approach to fertility regulation would be similar to that of the intrauterine device (IUD). This chapter will focus on the potential use of the first clinically available anti-progesterone, mifepristone (RU 486: Roussel-Uclaf), as a medical equivalent to the IUD.

Mifepristone is a 19-nor steroid with an affinity for the human progesterone receptor of about three times that of progesterone and an affinity for the glucocorticoid receptor of about two times that of dexamethasone. It has a lesser affinity for the androgen receptor and does not seem to interact with the oestrogen or mineralocorticoid receptors. Studies in rodents, rabbits and non-human primates have shown it to have potent anti-progesterone activity in vivo (Nieman and Loriaux, 1988). Thus mifepristone could, in theory, reduce or block progesterone action and prevent implantation. If effective, this would be an attractive strategy for birth control. In addition, the possibility remains that mifepristone would not disrupt a woman's normal hormonal patterns and would not involve ingestion of large amounts of exogenous steroids, as is currently the case with the available oral contraceptive agents.

From a practical perspective, many criteria must be satisfied before a drug can be used for this purpose. First, the dose–response effects on the menstrual cycle must be characterized. The optimal dose and schedule of administration should not alter the timing of the subsequent cycle, and the hormonal pattern of the subsequent cycle should be normal. This implies that the drug must have a short-lived ability to induce functional luteolysis coincident with menses, but it should not affect follicular development or the timing of ovulation in the next cycle. Ideally, the drug would be free of side-effects and toxicity, but, at the least, its toxicity must be known.

## DOSE–RESPONSE RELATIONSHIPS FOR MIFEPRISTONE

Hermann et al (1982) were the first to administer mifepristone in the luteal phase of the menstrual cycle. Three women received mifepristone for 4 days at a daily dose of 50 mg, beginning 7 days after the basal body temperature shift. All had menses within 48 h, resulting in a significant shortening of the cycle.

Nieman and co-workers (1985a,b) subsequently showed this same effect after a single mid-luteal phase dose of mifepristone. Eleven women were chosen for the study. All women used a non-hormonal birth control method during the study. Each had a history of regular menses (26–30 days). Mifepristone was given as a single mid luteal phase dose (2.5–25 mg/kg). All women who had a plasma progesterone level greater than 2.5 ng/ml and who received at least 5 mg/kg mifepristone had menses with 3 days of mifepristone administration. The subsequent menses occurred after a normal interval (26–30 days) in 6 of the 7 women. The seventh woman had an episode of bleeding 14 days after the mifepristone-induced menses. The hormonal data from her next cycle were consistent with disordered folliculogenesis and corpus luteum dysfunction. Subsequent cycles were normal.

Other investigators have confirmed that mifepristone can cause endometrial shedding when given during the luteal phase (Haspels, 1985; Schaison et al, 1985a; Croxatto et al, 1985, 1987; Nieman et al, 1987; Shoupe et al, 1987; van Santen and Haspels, 1987a,b; Yen et al, 1987). This effect is time-dependent. It occurs uniformly when the drug is given after the sixth luteal phase day, but not when given before the fifth luteal phase day (Table 1). As expected, there is no effect in anovulatory women (Schaison et al, 1985b). These data suggest that mifepristone effectively antagonizes progesterone action on well established secretory endometrium. The minimal dose of mifepristone required for this effect has not been established. A single mid luteal dose of roughly 1 mg/kg (as small as 50 mg) was effective in one study (Shoupe et al, 1987), while a daily dose of 0.5 mg/kg (25 mg) given for 4 days was effective only 80% of the time in another (Schaison et al, 1985a).

Luteolysis is seen most often when mifepristone is given in the mid to late luteal phase (Table 1). It is manifest as a decrease in plasma progesterone levels to concentrations seen in the follicular phase. Administration of mifepristone at a daily dose of approximately 1 mg/kg (50 mg) for 4 days given within 5 days of the luteinizing hormone (LH) surge caused luteolysis in three women (Hermann et al, 1985). A dose of 3 mg/kg given for 3 days was unsuccessful in eight women (Yen et al, 1987). Mid luteal phase administration of mifepristone resulted in luteolysis in 45% of women receiving

**Table 1.** Effects of luteal phase administration of mifepristone.

| Luteal phase day* | Mifepristone daily dose | Duration (days) | Post-mifepristone menses† | Interval menses† | Post-mifepristone luteolysis† | Next cycle | Reference |
|---|---|---|---|---|---|---|---|
| Day 4 | 50 mg | 4 | 1/3 | 0/3 | 3/3 | Normal | Hermann et al (1985) |
| Days 4–5 | 3 mg/kg | 3 | 8/8 | 8/8 | 0/8 | Short follicular phase | Yen et al (1987) |
| Day 7 | 10 mg/kg | 1 | 6/6 | 3/6 | 3/6 | Normal | Nieman et al (1987) |
| Day 7 | 2.5–25 mg/kg | 1 | 7/11 | 1/7 | 6/7 | Normal | Nieman et al (1985a) |
| Days 6–8 | 50 mg | 1 | 4/4 | 2/4 | 2/4 | Prolonged | Shoupe et al (1987) |
| Days 6–8 | 100 mg | 1 | 4/4 | 2/4 | 2/4 | Prolonged | Shoupe et al (1987) |
| Days 6–8 | 200 mg | 1 | 4/4 | 3/4 | 1/4 | Prolonged | Shoupe et al (1987) |
| Days 6–8 | 400 mg | 1 | 4/4 | 3/4 | 1/4 | Prolonged | Shoupe et al (1987) |
| Days 6–8 | 600 mg | 1 | 4/4 | 4/4 | 0/4 | Prolonged | Shoupe et al (1987) |
| Days 6–8 | 800 mg | 1 | 4/4 | 1/4 | 3/4 | Prolonged | Shoupe et al (1987) |
| Day 7 | 25 mg | 4 | 8/10 | 6/8 | 2/6 | Unknown | Schaison et al (1985a) |
| Day 7 | 50 mg | 4 | 7/8 | 4/7 | 3/7 | Unknown | Schaison et al (1985a) |
| Day 7 | 100 mg | 4 | 14/14 | 6/14 | 8/14 | Unknown | Schaison et al (1985a) |
| Day 8 | 50 mg | 4 | 4/4 | 0/4 | 4/4 | Normal | Hermann et al (1982) |
| Days 7–13 | 200 mg | 4 | 13/14 | 0/14 | 13/14 | Normal | Haspels (1985) |
| Days 9–13 | 100 mg | 4 | 6/6 | 0/6 | 6/6 | Prolonged follicular phase | Croxatto et al (1987) |
| Day 10 | 100 mg | 4 | 28/30 | 1/30 | 27/30 | Normal | Croxatto et al (1987) |
| Days 11–12 | 600 mg | 1 | 5/5 | 0/5 | 5/5 | Normal | Yen et al (1987) |

*Luteal phase day corresponds to the first day of mifepristone administration. It is expressed as the actual number of days after the luteinizing hormone surge or as calculated by the authors according to the day of the next expected menses.
†Expressed as the ratio of the number of responders to the number of pertinent cycles.

either single or multiple doses of the drug (Hermann et al, 1982; Nieman et al, 1985a, b, 1987; Schaison et al, 1985a; Croxatto et al, 1987; Shoupe et al, 1987). Mifepristone-induced regression of the corpus luteum in the mid luteal phase is dose-dependent when the drug is given on a 4-day schedule (Schaison et al, 1985a). Eight of 14 women showed luteolysis at a dose of 100 mg/day, while only 2 of 10 receiving 25 mg/day had complete luteolysis. Luteolysis was seen in all women (21/21) who received mifepristone in the late luteal phase, after cycle day 23 (Croxatto et al, 1987; Yen et al, 1987). Since luteolysis would be expected to occur after day 26 of a non-pregnant cycle, the occurrence of luteolysis cannot be unequivocally ascribed to mifepristone.

## EFFECTS OF LUTEAL PHASE ADMINISTRATION OF MIFEPRISTONE ON THE NEXT CYCLE

Ideally, treatment with mifepristone would not alter the timing or character of the menstrual cycle. While most studies have not addressed this issue directly, some pertinent information is available. In studies where luteolysis was linked to endometrial shedding, the length of the subsequent menstrual cycle was normal. This suggests that subsequent follicular development and ovulation were normal. The most direct, but usually least available, evidence for lack of effect on the subsequent cycle is documentation of a normal hormonal pattern in that cycle.

Luteolysis provides the best guide as to whether or not the subsequent cycle will be normal. Early luteal phase administration of the drug may decrease corpus luteum function without provoking endometrial shedding (Hermann et al, 1985; Croxatto et al, 1987). In this setting the treatment cycle may be prolonged as the ovarian events of the next cycle begin in the absence of menstrual bleeding. When mifepristone-induced luteolysis is incomplete, the hormonal pattern reflects continued but decreased corpus luteum function (Schaison et al, 1985a; Croxatto et al, 1987; Nieman et al, 1987; Shoupe et al, 1987; Yen et al, 1987). This presumably allows for transient renewed support of the endometrium, which is shed as progesterone levels decrease to the follicular phase range.

The subsequent cycle is generally normal when withdrawal bleeding is followed by luteolysis. While late luteal phase administration of the drug does not appear to alter subsequent menstrual cycle timing (Croxatto et al, 1987; Yen et al, 1987), very few women have been studied carefully at this time. The post-treatment cycle length in rhesus monkeys, however, is prolonged after parenteral administration of mifepristone in the late luteal phase (Shortle et al, 1985; Nieman et al, 1987). This phenomenon is dose-dependent and reflects an increase in follicular phase length. The difference between rhesus monkeys and man can probably be explained by differences in the pharmacokinetics of an orally administered dose compared to an intramuscular one. The day of administration (late compared with mid luteal) may also determine whether mifepristone can persist in the circulation at sufficiently high concentrations to affect the next follicular phase.

The plasma half-life of mifepristone after oral administration in men and women has been reported to be about 20–24 h (Heikinheimo et al, 1987; Kawai et al, 1987). This could play a role in subsequent cycles if the drug is given late enough in the luteal phase.

Croxatto and co-workers (1987) have investigated the effect of luteal phase administration of mifepristone for three successive cycles. Thirty cycles were investigated in ten women. All but three cycles were normal.

Continued support of the corpus luteum by human chorionic gonado-trophin (hCG) is an additional potential variable which might overcome the luteolytic effect of mifepristone and alter the timing of subsequent menses. This possibility has been evaluated by administering exogenous hCG in combination with mifepristone in the mid luteal phase (Croxatto et al, 1985; Nieman et al, 1987; Yen et al, 1987). When corpus luteum function was supported by exogenous hCG, luteal phase levels of progesterone persisted. Despite this, menses occurred in all women within 3 days. A second episode of bleeding occurred in most women within 20 days, and was coincident with a decrease in progesterone levels to < 2.5 ng/ml (8 mmol/l). This pattern of a second 'intermenstrual' bleeding episode was similar to that seen in women with incomplete luteolysis after mifepristone who did not receive hCG.

The way in which mifepristone impairs corpus luteum function is unclear. Exogenous hCG can block mifepristone induced luteolysis, suggesting that mifepristone-mediated luteolysis is mediated by inhibiting gonadotrophin secretion. Schaison and co-workers (1985a) have demonstrated a decrease in LH pulse amplitude in women given mifepristone during the luteal phase. Yen and co-workers (1987) have shown that this is a biphasic response, with an immediate increase and a subsequent decrease in LH pulse frequency within 24 h. These findings suggest that mifepristone has a progesterone-like (agonist) effect on gonadotrophin secretion. Others have described effects which also suggest that mifepristone is not a pure progesterone antagonist but can have mixed agonist–antagonist properties (Gravanis et al, 1985; Horwitz, 1985). Alternatively, the ability of mifepristone to inhibit steroido-genesis in granulosa cells in vitro suggests that direct inhibition of ovarian function by mifepristone could also contribute to regression of the corpus luteum (DiMattina et al, 1986).

## DOES LUTEAL PHASE ADMINISTRATION OF MIFEPRISTONE PREVENT PREGNANCY?

Mifepristone is an effective contraceptive in non-human primates. Given parenterally at a 5 mg/kg dose to female rhesus monkeys, mifepristone prevented pregnancy in 17 fecund cycles. Treatment with vehicle alone allowed pregnancy in 9 out of 32 fecund cycles ($P < 0.05$ by chi-squared analysis; Nieman et al, 1987). The drug is also effective when given to cynomolgus and female rhesus monkeys as a post-coital vaginal tampon (Hodgen, 1985).

The ability of mifepristone to prevent pregnancy has been tested in a limited number of women using either an occasional post-coital or a monthly luteal phase administration schedule, with mixed results (Haspels, 1985; Ulmann, 1987; van Santen and Haspels, 1987a,b).

## TOXICITY

Human toxicity data for mifepristone are limited. No adverse effects have been reported in healthy men and women following administration of the drug in single doses up to 25 mg/kg or daily total doses of 200 mg for 5 days (Hermann et al, 1982; Bertagna et al, 1984; Gaillard et al, 1984, 1985; Croxatto et al, 1985, 1987; Gravanis et al, 1985; Nieman et al, 1985a,b, 1987; Schaison et al, 1985a,b; Shoupe et al, 1987). Women treated for breast cancer at daily doses of 200 mg for up to 3 months had no adverse effects except for a mild to moderate decrease in the serum potassium level (Romieu et al, 1987). In contrast, Laue et al (1988) reported that 7 of 9 healthy men developed erythema multiforme after receiving daily doses of 10 mg/kg for 7 days. Liver, kidney, central nervous system and marrow toxicity have not been observed.

The anti-glucocorticoid effect of mifepristone in healthy men and women is seen at doses exceeding those required for an anti-progesterone effect, and is reversed by administration of a glucocorticoid such as dexamethasone. Mifepristone blocks cortisol negative feedback at the pituitary gland and induces a compensatory increase in plasma adrenocorticotrophic hormone and cortisol levels (Bertagna et al, 1984; Gaillard et al, 1984). The dose-dependent dissociation of anti-progesterone and anti-glucocorticoid activity and the compensatory increase in cortisol allow the drug to be used as an anti-progesterone without the risk of clinical adrenal insufficiency.

## SUMMARY

Mifepristone holds promise as a safe and effective anti-progesterone. Widespread use of mifepristone to regularize cycles or prevent pregnancy, however, cannot be recommended at this time. The drug is promising for these uses but the dose and timing of administration required to achieve optimum effect are unknown. Menses are consistently induced in the mid to late luteal phase at a wide range of doses. Further work needs to be done to examine the luteolytic properties of the drug when given at this time. Knowledge about the serum concentration of the parent compound and its less active metabolites after oral administration may help to explain variable biological effects. The effects of other modes of administration, such as transdermal or transvaginal application which avoid a first-pass effect by the liver, should also be explored.

Practical issues of the timing of administration need to be resolved. The drug is not effective when given in the absence of luteal phase levels of progesterone. Thus, verification of luteal phase status before the administration of the drug would be ideal. Basal body temperature monitoring may be one way to do this. There is no other convenient way to determine serum levels of progesterone that would be feasible on a large-scale outpatient basis. Since mifepristone does not regulate the timing of ovulation, the optimal time of administration may vary from cycle to cycle. This presumes a high degree of willingness on the part of the woman to observe her cycles and participate in decisions regarding the timing of the drug.

Mifepristone, the first clinically available anti-progesterone, represents a significant advance in fertility control. Further work is necessary to define the optimal dose and schedule of administration in the luteal phase and to explore the contraceptive efficacy in women at risk for pregnancy.

## REFERENCES

Bertagna X, Bertagna C, Luton JP, Husson JM & Girard F (1984) The new steroid analog RU 486 inhibits glucocorticoid action in man. *Journal of Clinical Endocrinology and Metabolism* **59:** 25–28.

Croxatto HB, Spitz IM, Salvatierra AM & Bardin CW (1985) The demonstration of the antiprogestin effects of RU 486 when administered to the human during hCG-induced pseudopregnancy. In Baulieu EE & Segal SJ (eds) *The Antiprogestin Steroid RU 486 and Human Fertility Control*, pp 263–269. New York: Plenum Press.

Croxatto HB, Salvatierra AM, Romero C & Spitz IM (1987) Late luteal phase administration of RU 486 for three successive cycles does not disrupt bleeding patterns or ovulation. *Journal of Clinical Endocrinology and Metabolism* **65:** 1272–1277.

DiMattina M, Albertson B, Saylor DE, Loriaux DL & Falk RJ (1986) Effect of the antiprogestin RU 486 on progesterone production by cultured human granulosa cells: inhibition of the ovarian 3α-hydroxysteroid dehydrogenase. *Contraception* **34:** 199–206.

Gaillard RC, Riondel A, Muller AF, Herrmann W & Baulieu EE (1984) RU 486: a steroid with antiglucocorticosteroid activity that only disinhibits the human pituitary–adrenal system at a specific time of day. *Proceedings of the National Academy of Science of the USA* **81:** 3879–3882.

Gaillard RC, Poffet D & Saurat JH (1985) RU 486 inhibits peripheral effects of glucocorticoids in humans. *Journal of Clinical Endocrinology and Metabolism* **61:** 1009–1011.

Gravanis A, Schaison G, George M et al (1985) Endometrial and pituitary responses to the steroidal antiprogestin RU 486 in postmenopausal women. *Journal of Clinical Endocrinology and Metabolism* **60:** 156–163.

Haspels AA (1985) Interruption of early pregnancy by the antiprogestational agent RU 486. In Baulieu EE & Segal SJ (eds) *The Antiprogestin Steroid RU 486 and Human Fertility Control*, pp 199–209. New York: Plenum Press.

Heikinheimo O, Lahteenmaki PLA, Koivunen E et al (1987) Metabolism and serum binding of RU 486 in women after various single doses. *Human Reproduction* **2:** 379–385.

Hermann W, Wyss R, Riondel A et al (1982) The effects of an antiprogesterone steroid in women: interruption of the menstrual cycle and early pregnancy. *Comptes Rendus de l'Académie des Sciences de Paris* (III) **294:** 933–938.

Hermann WL, Schindler AM, Wyss R & Bischof P (1985) Effects of the antiprogesterone RU 486 in early pregnancy and during the menstrual cycle. In Baulieu EE & Segal SJ (eds) *The Antiprogestin Steroid RU 486 and Human Fertility Control*, pp 179–198. New York: Plenum Press.

Hodgen GD (1985) Pregnancy prevention by intravaginal delivery of a progesterone antagonist: RU 486 tampon for menstrual induction and absorption. *Fertility and Sterility* **44:** 263–267.

Horwitz KB (1985) The antiprogestin RU 38486: receptor-mediated progestin versus antiprogestin actions screened in estrogen-insensitive T47D$_{co}$ human breast cancer cells. *Endocrinology* **116:** 2236–2245.

Kawai S, Nieman LK, Brandon DD, Udelsman R, Loriaux DL & Chrousos GP (1987) Pharmacokinetic properties of the glucocorticoid and progesterone antagonist RU 486 in man. *Journal of Pharmacology and Experimental Therapeutics* **241:** 401–406.

Laue L, Barnes K & Fleisher T (1988) Effects of chronic hypercortisolism and hypocortisolism on leukocyte subpopulations. *Endocrinology* **122 (supplement):** 213.

Nieman LK & Loriaux DL (1988) Clinical applications of the glucocorticoid and progestin antagonist RU 486. In Agarwal MK (ed) *Receptor Mediated Antisteroid Action*, pp 77–97. Berlin: Walter de Gruyter.

Nieman LK, Healy DL, Spitz IM et al (1985a) Induction of menses in normal women by a single dose of the antiprogesterone steroid RU 486. *Clinical Research* **33:** 312A.

Nieman LK, Healy DL, Spitz IM et al (1985b) Use of single doses of the antiprogesterone steroid RU 486 for induction of menstruation in normal women. In Baulieu EE & Segal SJ (eds) *The Antiprogestin Steroid RU 486 and Human Fertility Control*, pp 279–283. New York: Plenum Press.

Nieman LK, Choate TM, Chrousos GP et al (1987) The progesterone antagonist RU 486: a potential new contraceptive agent. *New England Journal of Medicine* **316:** 187–191.

Romieu G, Maudelonde T, Ulmann A et al (1987) The antiprogestin RU 486 in advanced breast cancer: preliminary clinial trial. *Bulletin of Cancer (Paris)* **74:** 455–461.

Schaison G, George M, Lestrat N, Reinberg A & Baulieu EE (1985a) Effects of the anti-progesterone steroid RU 486 during mid luteal phase in normal women. *Journal of Clinical Endocrinology and Metabolism* **61:** 484–489.

Schaison G, Lestrat N, Couzinet B, deBrux J, Bouchard P & Baulieu EE (1985b) Effects of the antiprogestin steroid RU 486 in women with anovulatory cycles. *Endocrinology* **116 (supplement):** 156.

Shortle B, Dyrenfurth I & Ferin M (1985) Effects of an antiprogesterone agent, RU 486, on the menstrual cycle of the rhesus monkey. *Journal of Clinical Endocrinology and Metabolism* **60:** 731–735.

Shoupe D, Mishell DR, Lahteenmaki P et al (1987) Effects of the antiprogesterone RU 486 in normal women. *American Journal of Obstetrics and Gynecology* **157:** 1415–1420.

Ulmann A (1987) Uses of RU 486 for contragestion: an update. *Contraception* **36 (supplement):** 21–31.

van Santen MR & Haspels AA (1987a) Interception III: postcoital luteal contragestion by an antiprogestin (mifepristone, RU 486) in 62 women. *Contraception* **35:** 423–431.

van Santen MR & Haspels AA (1987b) Interception IV: failure of mifepristone (RU 486) as a monthly contragestive, Lunarette. *Contraception* **35:** 433–443.

Yen S, Garzo G & Liu J (1987) Luteal contraception. *Contraception* **36 (supplement):** 13–25.

# 7

## Anti-progesterones for the interruption of pregnancy

M. BYGDEMAN
P. F. A. VAN LOOK

### INTRODUCTION

Progesterone is a key hormone in the establishment and maintenance of human pregnancy. An antiprogesterone drug would therefore induce menstruation when administered in the luteal phase of the menstrual cycle, prevent implantation when administered at nidation and induce abortion when administered in early pregnancy.

The object of the present article is to summarize the experience obtained so far in the clinical application of this type of drug to terminate pregnancy. The first drug to be used for this purpose was RU 486 (mifepristone, Roussel Uclaf, Paris; Baulieu, 1985). More recently, compounds ZK 98.734 and ZK 98.299, with a similar action have been developed by Schering AG, Berlin (Wiechert and Neef, 1987). While these compounds act as antiprogesterones at the receptor level, Epostane (WIN 32.729, Sterling-Winthrop, Guildford, UK) is a progesterone synthesis inhibitor which exerts its effect by inhibiting the $3\beta$-hydroxysteroid dehydrogenase enzyme system (Rabe et al, 1983).

### Termination of early pregnancy by antiprogesterones alone

#### Mifepristone

In the first clinical study on the effect of mifepristone in early pregnancy Herrmann and associates (1982) demonstrated that oral administration of 200 mg/day of the compound for 4 days to women who were 6–8 weeks pregnant induced abortion in 9 of 11 patients. Of the 9 patients one had an incomplete abortion. Shortly thereafter, a collaborative study by the World Health Organization was established in which the antiprogesterone was given to 37 women seeking termination of pregnancy at an amenorrhoea of 42 days or less (Kovacs et al, 1984). These patients were given 25, 50 or 100 mg mifepristone twice daily for 4 days. Twenty-two patients had a complete abortion (61%) while 11 had an incomplete abortion. Of the remaining four patients one had an extrauterine pregnancy and in the other three the treatment failed. There were no differences in success rate between the different dose schedules.

In later studies the dose of mifepristone has been increased but the duration of treatment kept unchanged. Couzinet et al (1986) reported a success rate between 82.4 and 88.5% in women with a menstrual delay of ten days or less if the daily dose was 100 or 150 mg. Vervest and Haspels reported (1985) a success rate of 83% using 100 or 200 mg daily and Elia (1985) had a complete abortion rate of 39% with 200 mg. Shoupe et al (1986), on the other hand, reported only one patient with complete abortion out of 10 women given a daily dose of 200 or 400 mg.

A longer duration of treatment has been evaluated by several investigators (Table 1). Mishell et al (1987) used either 50 or 100 mg daily for 7 days and reported a frequency of complete abortion of 50 and 73%, respectively, while Birgerson and Odlind (1987) with the same dose schedules found a success rate of 61% in both treatment groups.

Table 1. Termination of early pregnancy by mifepristone alone.

| Mifepristone daily dose (mg) | Duration of treatment (days) | Duration of amenorrhoea (days) | Frequency of complete abortion (%) | Reference |
|---|---|---|---|---|
| 200 | 4 | 42–56 | 73 | Herrmann et al, 1982 |
| 50 100 200 | 4 | up to 42 | 61 | Kovacs et al, 1984 |
| 50 100 | 7 7 | up to 49 up to 49 | 50 73 | Mishell et al, 1987 |
| 50 100 | 7 7 | up to 49 up to 49 | 61 61 | Birgerson and Odlind, 1987 |
| 400 | 2 | up to 38 | 85 | Couzinet et al, 1986 |
| 600 600 | 1 1 | up to 41 over 42 | 84 58 | Ulmann, 1987 |

Another treatment approach has been to use a high dose of mifepristone but to restrict the duration of treatment to 1 or 2 days. A daily dose of 400 mg mifepristone for 2 days resulted in a frequency of complete abortion of 85% (Couzinet et al, 1986) and following a single dose of 600 mg the success rate varied between 84% if the duration of amenorrhoea was less than 41 days and 58% if the duration of amenorrhoea was more than 42 days (Ulmann, 1987).

Thus, the clinical data indicate that if mifepristone is used alone during early pregnancy the compound is capable of inducing a complete abortion in approximately 60% of the patients (range 10–87%). Neither the size of individual dose nor the duration of treatment seems to have a significant influence on the outcome of therapy.

It is at present entirely unclear why some women fail to respond to treatment with mifepristone. In several studies the successfully treated patients were compared with those in whom the treatment failed. No consistent relation has been found, however, between treatment outcome and physical characteristics or hormone levels of the subjects at the start of treatment. In the study of Kovacs (1985) and that of Elia (1985), successfully treated women tended to have lower levels of oestradiol but this was not confirmed by Shoupe et al (1986) who reported instead a tendency towards lower human chorionic gonadotrophin (hCG) and progesterone levels in their successful cases. Significantly lower pretreatment β-hCG and progesterone levels were also found by Mishell et al (1987) in women who aborted than in those who did not but the difference was only present in one of their two treatment groups. Moreover, Couzinet et al (1986) did not find pretreatment levels of oestradiol, progesterone and β-hCG to be predictive of treatment outcome. The plasma levels of mifepristone in successfully and unsuccessfully treated patients have also been compared but no differences have been found (Couzinet et al, 1986; Mishell et al, 1987).

The only parameter which seems to be related to the outcome of treatment is duration of pregnancy. In general, in the studies reporting a high success rate of around 85%, only patients with a menstrual delay of up to 14 days were treated (Couzinet et al, 1986; Ulmann, 1987). When pregnancy is somewhat more advanced (up to 56 days of amenorrhoea) the average rate of complete abortion that can be calculated from trials published to date is 63% (Van Look, 1988). The reason for this difference is also unclear but it is possible that, since in early pregnancy progesterone originates mostly from the corpus luteum and its plasma concentration is relatively low, it can be more effectively antagonized by mifepristone than in slightly more advanced pregnancy when implantation is better established and the placenta produces a considerable local amount of progesterone.

*Epostane*

The clinical experience with epostane for termination of early pregnancy is more limited than that for mifepristone. Birgerson and Odlind (1987) have reported that treatment with 200 mg epostane four times a day for 7 days resulted in successful termination of pregnancy in 73% of the patients, indicating that the effectiveness of this type of therapy is approximately the same as that of mifepristone during early pregnancy.

*ZK 98.734 and ZK 98.299*

Both these compounds have been shown capable of inducing abortion in the guinea-pig. Most effective was ZK 98.734. With this compound all animals aborted following 30 mg administered subcutaneously for 2 days compared to 7/9 animals and 4/9 animals, respectively, if the same dose of ZK 98.299 and mifepristone was used (Elger et al, 1987). ZK 98.734 has reached the initial phase of clinical testing but no results have so far been published.

**Sequential therapy of antiprogesterone and prostaglandin for termination of early pregnancy**

*Experimental studies*

The contractility of the pregnant human uterus is believed to be hormonally regulated. During early human pregnancy uterine activity is suppressed and the inactivity may be due to a blocking effect of progesterone (Csapo, 1970). A decrease in plasma progesterone following lutectomy in early pregnancy was associated with an increased myometrial sensitivity to prostaglandin (Csapo et al, 1973). The fact that treatment with mifepristone during early pregnancy resulted in an increased uterine contractility was first demonstrated by Bygdeman and Swahn (1985). In a more extensive study (Swahn and Bygdeman, 1988) it was shown that treatment with 25 mg mifepristone twice daily resulted in the appearance of regular uterine contractions at 24 h in two of five patients and in all patients 36 h, 48 h and 72 h after the start of mifepristone treatment. Intramuscular administration of the prostaglandin (PG) analogue, 16-phenoxy-tetranor $PGE_2$ methyl sulphonylamide (Sulprostone, Schering AG, Berlin) to control patients who had not been pretreated with mifepristone, led to an increase in uterine tonus upon which irregular contractions of low amplitude were superimposed. The uterine response to sulprostone was dose-related. After pretreatment with mifepristone the uterine response to the $PGE_2$ analogue was qualitatively and quantitatively different from that in the control group. The sensitivity of the myometrium significantly increased and the contractions, superimposed on the increased uterine tonus, were more co-ordinated. The increase in sensitivity to the prostaglandin was already apparent 24 h after the start of mifepristone treatment. Doses as low as 0.05 mg of the PGE-analogue had a marked stimulatory effect on uterine contractility (Figure 1).

Increased sensitivity of the uterus after mifepristone treatment has also been demonstrated for 16,16-dimethyl-trans-$\Delta^2$ $PGE_1$ methyl ester (Gemeprost, May & Baker, Dagenham, UK) administered vaginally in a dose of 1.0 mg

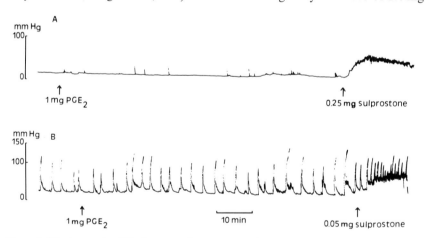

**Figure 1.** Uterine contractility in two early pregnant patients.

**Patient A** has received no pretreatment and the uterus is inactive. There is no response to oral administration of 1.0 mg $PGE_2$ while an intramuscular injection of 0.25 mg sulprostone resulted in an increase in uterine tonus with irregular contractions superimposed.

**Patient B** has been pretreated with 25 mg mifepristone twice daily for 48 h. Regular uterine contractions have developed and the sensitivity to sulprostone has increased but there is still no effect of oral $PGE_2$.

(Swahn and Bygdeman, unpublished observations), but oral doses of 1.0–1.5 mg $PGE_2$ were without effect under the same experimental conditions (Swahn et al, 1988). Interestingly, treatment with mifepristone did not influence the sensitivity to oxytocin (Swahn and Bygdeman, 1988).

Following treatment with epostane in different doses, 300–600 mg daily for 5 days, vaginal administration of 10 mg $PGE_2$ in suppository form to patients in early pregnancy resulted in an increased uterine contractility but only in patients in whom progesterone had decreased markedly (Webster et al, 1985). These results lend support to the hypothesis that progesterone has a determining influence on the sensitivity of the myometrium to prostaglandins.

In the pregnant guinea-pig the abortifacient effect of mifepristone and of ZK 98.299 was significantly enhanced by the addition of a low dose of sulprostone, indicating that antiprogesterones sensitize the myometrium to prostaglandins in this species also. However, this may not be a general rule since neither the abortion rate nor the abortion–induction interval was favourably influenced by sulprostone in animals treated with ZK 98.734 (Elger et al, 1986).

## Clinical results

The efficacy of mifepristone given in combination with different prostaglandins for termination of early pregnancy has been evaluated in several clinical studies (Table 2). In the first study 25 mg mifepristone was given twice daily for 4 days. In the morning of the fourth day 0.25 mg sulprostone was administered as an intramuscular injection (Bygdeman and Swahn, 1985). The combined treatment resulted in complete abortion in 32 out of 34 patients (94%). One patient experienced an incomplete abortion and in one patient the pregnancy continued unaffected. The number of patients was subsequently increased to 74, of whom 71 (96%) aborted completely, further supporting the concept that a combined treatment of mifepristone and sulprostone is more effective than mifepristone alone (Swahn and Bygdeman, 1987).

**Table 2.** Termination of early pregnancy by mifepristone in combination with prostaglandin analogues.

| Mifepristone daily dose (mg) | Type of prostaglandin and dose (mg) | Duration of amenorrhoea (days) | Frequency of complete abortion (%) | Reference |
|---|---|---|---|---|
| 50 | Sulprostone 0.25 | up to 49 | 96 | Bygdeman & Swahn, 1985; Swahn & Bygdeman, 1987 |
| 150 | Gemeprost 1.0 | up to 56 | 95 | Cameron et al, 1986 |
| 150 400 500 single dose 600 | Gemeprost 0.5 or 1.0 | up to 56 | 95 | Rodger and Baird, 1987 |
| 600 single dose | Gemeprost 1.0 | up to 49 | 100 | Dubois et al, 1988 |

Mifepristone has also been combined with vaginal administration of gemeprost. In a randomized study including 39 patients in early pregnancy, 19 women received only mifepristone (150 mg daily for 4 days). The remainder were given the same mifepristone regimen but in addition received 1 mg gemeprost 48 h after commencing the antiprogesterone therapy. The combined treatment was found to be significantly more effective (18/19 had complete abortion) than if mifepristone was given alone (12/20 complete abortion; Cameron et al, 1986).

In a second study 100 women in early pregnancy were treated with either 150 mg mifepristone daily for 4 days or with a single administration of 400, 500 or 600 mg mifepristone followed in all patients by a 1 mg gemeprost suppository, either as a single dose or divided into two, and given with a 3–6-h interval 48 h after the initiation of mifepristone therapy. The second half of the gemeprost suppository was given only if there was no uterine pain or bleeding. The effectiveness of the four treatment regimens was similar. There were no on-going pregnancies and 95 of the 100 women aborted completely. Of the 74 women who received half a gemeprost suppository (0.5 mg) only 10 (14%) required the second half (Rodger and Baird, 1987). The fact that the combination of a single dose of 600 mg mifepristone and 1 mg gemeprost is an effective method to terminate early pregnancy has been further supported by a French multicentre study on 106 women with an amenorrhoea of up to 49 days. In this study all patients aborted completely following treatment (Dubois et al, 1988).

Mifepristone has also been combined with oral $PGE_2$ in a double-blind randomized controlled efficacy trial. The treatment was 25 mg mifepristone twice daily for 4 days and 1 mg $PGE_2$ or placebo once or twice on the last day of mifepristone therapy. The results indicated that oral $PGE_2$ at the doses employed did not improve the rate of complete abortion achieved with mifepristone and thus oral $PGE_2$, when given in clinically acceptable doses, is not a suitable alternative to synthetic PGE analogues for use in combination with mifepristone for termination of early pregnancy (Swahn et al, 1988).

It is interesting to note that addition of ergonovine 0.2 mg six times with 4 h interval (Mishell et al, 1987) or oxytocin (Ulmann, personal communication) did not increase the frequency of complete abortion in comparison with mifepristone alone.

Epostane treatment in combination with vaginal administration of $PGE_2$ for termination of early pregnancy was reported by Webster et al (1985). The study included 20 women consecutively assigned to four treatment groups. The first group was treated with 10 mg $PGE_2$ in vaginal suppositories three times at 2-h intervals. The three remaining groups received 300, 400 or 600 mg epostane daily for 5 days and were treated with the same dose of $PGE_2$ on the fourth day. Abortion was induced in one of the five patients receiving only $PGE_2$, in three of ten patients treated with the two lowest doses of epostane and in all five patients receiving 600 mg epostane plus $PGE_2$. The highest dose of epostane was associated with the greatest decline in progesterone and oestradiol.

## Bleeding pattern

Almost all patients start to bleed following treatment with mifepristone. The frequency of non-responders varies slightly between studies but with daily doses of 50 mg or more mifepristone it is usually around 2% (Ulmann, 1987). The majority of the patients started to bleed on the second or third day of treatment (Kovacs et al, 1984; Mishell et al, 1987; Ulmann, 1987; Swahn et al, 1988). The successfully treated patients tended to start bleeding earlier than the failures (Mishell et al, 1987) and the start of bleeding also seemed to be dose-related (Kovacs et al, 1984; Mishell et al, 1987; Birgerson and Odlind, 1987).

The mean duration of bleeding in successful cases was approximately 1–2 weeks and in failures significantly shorter, or less than 1 week. Couzinet et al (1986), for instance, reported a mean duration of bleeding in successes of $11.6 \pm 5.8$ days compared to $3.4 \pm 1.7$ days in failures. In the study of Mishell et al (1987) the corresponding values were 13.5–14.7 days and 7.3–9.2 days depending on the dose of mifepristone used; in the study of Swahn et al (1988) values were $16.8 \pm 2.0$ and $7.8 \pm 1.0$ days, respectively. The longer duration of bleeding in the successfully treated patients in this study was ascribed by these authors to the more advanced stage of pregnancy at the time of treatment than in the study of Couzinet et al (1986).

The amount of blood loss has been reported to be relatively heavy; greater than a normal menses and more compatible with miscarriage-related metrorrhagia. In successful cases the overall blood loss measured quantitatively was $87 \pm 9$ ml according to Kovacs (1985) and 53 ml (range 2–227 ml) according to Cameron et al (1986), or approximately 50% more than that of a normal menstruation.

Excessive bleeding has been reported in several studies. The frequency varied between 0% (Couzinet et al, 1986) to 5.6% (Kovacs et al, 1984). In French clinical trials comprising 1500 women six subjects (0.4%) had to have a blood transfusion (Ulmann, 1987).

In the study of Birgerson and Odlind (1987) in which epostane and mifepristone were compared, patients treated with mifepristone started to bleed significantly earlier (1–2 days) than those who were given epostane. Otherwise the bleeding patterns after both treatments were similar.

The bleeding pattern following treatment with mifepristone and different PG analogues seems, with regard to start of bleeding, duration of bleeding and amount of blood loss, to be the same as with mifepristone alone. It is possible that the risk of excessive bleeding is reduced after the combined therapy. In approximately 300 women treated with mifepristone and prostaglandin analogues, this complication has not been reported to date but the number of women is not yet large enough to permit estimation of the excessive bleeding risk with such combination regimens (Bygdeman and Swahn, 1985; Cameron et al, 1986; Rodger and Baird, 1987; Swahn and Bygdeman, 1987; Dubois et al, 1988).

## Side-effects

Side-effects during treatment with mifepristone were generally of a mild nature and similar in all clinical studies. Most commonly reported were nausea, vomiting, fatigue, headache and contractions that were more painful than normal menstrual pain during the passage of the abortion products. All these side-effects, except for abdominal pain, are common during pregnancy. It is therefore interesting to note that in the study of Swahn et al (1988) in which the occurrence of nausea, vomiting, dizziness and fatigue was recorded daily before and during mifepristone treatment, there was no significant increase in the frequency of these side-effects during the treatment days. Abdominal pain, on the other hand, was reported by 7% of the patients prior to treatment as compared to 43% on the fourth treatment day. Similar results have also been reported by Cameron et al (1986).

The incidence of pregnancy-related side-effects does not seem to be higher if mifepristone and PG analogues are used in combination (Bygdeman and Swahn, 1985; Cameron et al, 1986). Cameron et al (1986) reported that the frequency of abdominal pain did not differ significantly between the patients who received mifepristone alone or in combination with 1 mg gemeprost. Only three women in this study required pethidine or diamorphine for pain relief; all three belonged, however, to the group receiving the combined treatment. It is our experience also that strong uterine pain is more frequent (5–10%) when PG analogues are added and that it generally occurs at the time of PG treatment (Bygdeman and Swahn, 1985; Swahn and Bygdeman, 1987).

In doses with similar efficacy, nausea sometimes associated with vomiting occurred significantly more often during treatment with epostane (800 mg daily) than with mifepristone (50 or 100 mg daily; Birgerson and Odlind, 1987).

## Effect on plasma hormone levels

Mifepristone acts as an antagonist not only to progesterone but also to glucocorticoids at the receptor level (Baulieu, 1985). In the cynomolgus monkey Healy et al (1985) have demonstrated both a dose- and time-dependent increase in plasma adrenocorticotrophic hormone (ACTH), cortisol and arginine vasopressin following treatment with mifepristone.

Most of the clinical studies to date in which ACTH and/or cortisol have been measured have shown an increased plasma concentration of these hormones during treatment with mifepristone (Kovacs et al, 1984; Kovacs, 1985; Couzinet et al, 1986; Shoupe et al, 1986; Swahn et al, 1988). An exception is Mishell et al (1987) who did not find an increase in cortisol on day 4 in pregnant women treated with 25 mg mifepristone twice daily for 7 days. In the study by Kovacs et al (1984) a moderate increase in plasma cortisol was found with 25 mg mifepristone twice daily. If the dose was increased to 50 or 100 mg twice daily no further elevation of plasma cortisol levels was observed, indicating that at least part of the increase could be due to a stress response to the abortion itself. The increase in cortisol levels also depends on the time of mifepristone administration. A single dose of 400 mg mifepristone administered at 02.00 h elevated plasma cortisols from 07.00 h until 12.00 h. In contrast, administration of the same dose at 14.00 h produced no significant rise in plasma cortisol (Bertagna et al, 1984). Since mifepristone-induced blockade of the glucocorticoid receptor could increase the risk for complications during anaesthesia and surgery, for instance in patients needing curettage, it is important to note that in all studies published to date the cortisol rise has been modest and that mean levels have not exceeded the normal range.

Beside ACTH and cortisol, an increase in prolactin has been observed during mifepristone treatment (Swahn et al, 1988). In the same study levels of aldosterone tended to be slightly higher on the second day of a 4-day treatment with mifepristone (25 mg twice daily) but the increase was not sustained in spite of persistently elevated cortisol.

Plasma levels of progesterone, 17β-oestradiol and β-hCG showed similar profiles during mifepristone treatment. In successfully treated patients β-hCG and progesterone concentrations remained essentially unchanged while 17β-oestradiol concentration increased slightly during the first 2–3 days following the start of mifepristone treatment. Thereafter, the levels of the three hormones declined rapidly and were significantly lower than pretreatment levels 1 week after initiation of mifepristone therapy (Kovacs et al, 1984; Kovacs, 1985; Mishell et al, 1987; Swahn et al, 1988). The decline of β-hCG seemed somewhat slower than that of the steroid hormones. In the study of Kovacs et al (1984), in which different doses of mifepristone were administered during 4 days, the rate of decline of all three hormones was dose-related. In failure patients, the levels of 17β-oestradiol, progesterone and β-hCG remained at or above pretreatment levels. Thus, on days 4 to 7 the concentration of these hormones was significantly lower in successfully treated subjects than in failure cases, as also reported by Mishell et al (1987) and Swahn et al (1988).

## Mode of action

The mechanism by which mifepristone interrupts early pregnancy is not clear. Blockage of progesterone action at its receptor sites is probably the first in a series of events that leads to decidual necrosis, bleeding, separation of the conceptus and eventually to the expulsion of the products of conception. Histological studies in women have shown that, although mifepristone induced decidual necrosis, it caused no significant alterations of the tropho-blast (Herrmann et al, 1985). The fact that plasma β-hCG remains relatively constant during the first days of mifepristone treatment and does not decline dramatically until abortion suggests that mifepristone does not affect pregnancy through a direct effect on β-hCG secretion. The decline in β-hCG is most likely the result of trophoblast separation. Since the levels of plasma progesterone and oestradiol also remain essentially unchanged initially, it is also unlikely that mifepristone has a primary luteolytic effect in early pregnancy.

Blockage of the progesterone receptors and the resulting withdrawal of progesterone at the cellular level probably causes a number of local events, as discussed by Healy (1985). Of special interest are the prostaglandins $PGF_{2\alpha}$ and $PGE_2$. Smith and Kelly (1987) incubated enriched preparations of glandular and stromal cells obtained from early human decidua with mifepristone and ZK 98.734 for 24 h. The results suggested that the anti-progesterones stimulated the synthesis of both prostaglandins by glandular cells through an effect on cyclo-oxygenase activity. On the other hand, in vivo studies in the guinea-pig indicated that intrauterine administration of the antiprogesterone ZK 98.299 inhibited the release of $PGF_{2\alpha}$ from the endometrium as judged from the occurrence of delayed luteal regression (Elger et al, 1988) Csapo (1974) has proposed that the degree of uterine activity during pregnancy is regulated by the balance between the intrinsic suppressor, progesterone, and the stimulant, $PGF_{2\alpha}$. The observed increase in uterine contractility following mifepristone treatment (Bygdeman and Swahn, 1985; Swahn and Bygdeman, 1988) could, thus, be due to an increased endogenous prostaglandin production. It is possible, however, that the withdrawal of progesterone blockage could be sufficient to cause the change in uterine contractility and the increased sensitivity of the myometrium to prostaglandins without any substantial increase in endogenous prostaglandin production. In spontaneous abortion it is believed that an increase in the endogenous production of prostaglandins plays an essential role in the abortion process. The increase in the frequency of complete abortions, observed when treatment with mifepristone is complemented by administration of PG analogues, indicates that local withdrawal of progesterone influence may not be an equally effective trigger of PG production as the factors regulating an early spontaneous abortion.

The appearance of gap junctions between myometrial cells, which is accompanied by an increase in the ability of spontaneous and evoked electrical activity to propagate between myometrial cells, is essential for co-ordinated uterine contractility during labour. Progesterone inhibits gap junctions in all models studied (see Garfield, 1984). Thus, it is possible that the regular contractility pattern and the change in response to PG observed after mifepristone therapy may be due to a mifepristone -induced development of gap junctions (see Garfield and Baulieu, 1987).

### Other clinical applications

In the pregnant guinea-pig, treatment with mifepristone ZK 98.734 and ZK 98.299 resulted in a marked softening and dilatation of the cervix (Elger et al, 1986). In the human the effect does not seem equally impressive. Following oral administration of 100 mg mifepristone 24 and 12 h prior to vacuum aspiration, the degree of cervical dilatation was not significantly different from that following placebo. However, quantitation of the force needed to introduce increasing sizes of Hegar probes to dilate further the cervical canal indicated a lower cervical resistance in the group of patients receiving mifepristone than in controls (Rådestad et al, 1988).

Prostaglandins are often used to terminate second-trimester pregnancy. In a recent study, 40 patients with viable pregnancies of 16–18 weeks' gestation were treated with extra-amniotic infusion of $PGE_2$ in incremental doses. Twenty of the patients were pretreated with a single dose of 200 mg mifepristone 24 h before starting the PG infusion. A significant reduction in both the induction-to-abortion interval and the total dose of PG needed to induce abortion was observed in the mifepristone-treated group (Urquhart and Templeton, 1987).

## SUMMARY

Therapeutic abortion can be performed effectively and safely by vacuum aspiration of the uterus up to 12 weeks of amenorrhoea. Although the operative procedure could be regarded as simple, complications do occur and attempts have been made to develop non-surgical means of terminating pregnancy in the first 3–4 weeks following the first missed menstrual period. A variety of PG analogues have been developed which induce abortion in over 90% of women when given by vaginal pessary or intramuscular injections (see Bygdeman, 1984). In a large multicentre study (WHO, 1987) 0.5 mg sulprostone, administered three times with 3 h intervals, was recently found to be equally as effective as vacuum aspiration for termination of early pregnancy. The frequencies of complete abortion were 91 and 94%, respectively. However, the widespread acceptance of PG treatment is limited by a relatively high incidence of gastrointestinal side-effects and uterine pain.

Treatment with antiprogesterones, both mifepristone and epostane, effectively induces abortion during early pregnancy, but the frequency of complete abortion is too low to be clinically acceptable. It remains to be demonstrated if other antiprogesterones such as ZK 98.734 and ZK 98.299, currently under development, may change this conclusion.

Administration of mifepristone induces uterine contractions and increases the sensitivity of the myometrium to prostaglandins. These effects allowed the development of sequential treatment with a low dose of mifepristone and PG analogues administered vaginally or intramuscularly. The combined therapy has been shown to be highly effective (frequency of complete abortion between 95 and 100%) and is seemingly associated with a lower frequency of side-effects than if PG analogues are used alone. Whether this medical abortion method will be a realistic alternative to vacuum aspiration during the first 8 weeks of pregnancy depends on the outcome of further clinical trials, including randomized studies comparing the two procedures. It has been shown that mifepristone crosses the placenta (Frydman et al, 1985). An important factor which needs to be verified in future studies is therefore the possible embryotoxicity of this type of compound. The risk that pregnancy continues in spite of treatment can never be excluded.

It is conceivable that antiprogesterones may also be used in the future to soften the cervix and dilate the cervical canal prior to vacuum aspiration in late first-trimester and early second-trimester pregnancy and to induce second-trimester abortion or potentiate the uterine effect of other drugs, such as prostaglandins and hypertonic saline, presently in use for this purpose.

# REFERENCES

Baulieu EE (1985) RU 486: an antiprogestin steroid with contragestive activity in women. In Baulieu EE & Segal SJ (eds) *The Antiprogestin Steroid RU 486 and Human Fertility Control*, pp 1–25. New York: Plenum Press.

Bertagna X, Bertagna C, Luton JP, Husson JM & Girard F (1984) The new steroid analog RU 486 inhibits glucocorticoid action in man. *Journal of Clinical Endocrinology and Metabolism* 59: 25–28.

Birgerson L & Odlind V (1987) Early pregnancy termination with antiprogestins: a comparative clinical study of RU 486 given in two dose regimens and epostane. *Fertility and Sterility* 48: 565–570.

Bygdeman M (1984) The use of prostaglandins and their analogues for abortion. *Clinics in Obstetrics and Gynaecology* 11: 573–584.

Bygdeman M & Swahn ML (1985) Progesterone receptor blockage. Effect on uterine contractility and early pregnancy. *Contraception* 32: 45–51.

Cameron IT, Michie AF & Baird DT (1986) Therapeutic abortion in early pregnancy with antiprogestogen RU 486 alone or in combination with prostaglandin analogue (gemeprost). *Contraception* 34: 459–468.

Couzinet B, LeStrat N, Ulmann A, Baulieu EE & Schaison G (1986) Termination of early pregnancy by the progesterone antagonist RU 486 (mifepristone). *New England Journal of Medicine* 315: 1565–1570.

Csapo AI (1970) The diagnostic significance of the intrauterine pressure. *Obstetrical and Gynecological Survey* 25: 515–543.

Csapo AI (1974) 'Prostaglandin impact' for menstrual induction. *Population Reports, Series G* 4: G33–G40.

Csapo AI, Pulkkinen MO & Kaihola HL (1973) The effect of lutectomy induced progesterone withdrawal on the oxytocin and prostaglandin response of the first trimester pregnant human uterus. *Prostaglandins* 4: 421–429.

Dubois C, Ulmann A, Aubeny E et al (1988) Contragestion par le RU 486: intérêt de l'association à un dérivé prostaglandine. *Comptes Rendus de l'Académie des Sciences, Paris*, 306: 57–61.

Elger W, Beier S, Chwalisz K et al (1986) Studies on the mechanisms of action of progesterone antagonists. *Journal of Steroid Biochemistry* 25: 835–845.

Elger W, Fahnrich M, Beier S, Qing SS & Chwalisz (1987) Endometrial and myometrial effects of progesterone antagonists in pregnant guinea pigs. *American Journal of Obstetrics and Gynecology* 157(Supplement): 1065–1074.

Elger W, Esch A, Fahnrich M et al (1988) Antiluteolytic effects of progesterone antagonists (AG) in the cyclic guinea pig are due to inhibition of uterine prostaglandin (PG) synthesis or liberation. *Acta Endocrinologica* Supplement 287: 40–41.

Elia D (1985) Clinical study of RU 486 in early pregnancy. In Baulieu EE & Segal SJ (eds) *The Antiprogestin Steroid RU 486 and Human Fertility Control*, pp 211–220. New York: Plenum Press.

Frydman R, Taylor S & Ulmann A (1985) Transplacental passage of mifepristone. *Lancet* ii: 1252.

Garfield RE (1984) Control of myometrial junction in preterm versus term labor. *Clinical Obstetrics and Gynecology* 27: 572–591.

Garfield RE & Baulieu EE (1987) The antiprogesterone steroid RU 486: a short pharmacological and clinical review, with emphasis on the interruption of pregnancy. *Clinical Endocrinology and Metabolism, Reproductive Endocrinology* 1(1): 207–221.

Healy DL (1985) Clinical status of antiprogesterone steroids. *Clinical Reproduction and Fertility* 3: 277–296.

Healy DL, Chrousos GP, Schulte HM, Gold PW & Hodgen GD (1985) Increased adrenocorticotropin, cortisol and arginine vasopressin secretion in primates after the antiglucocorticoid steroid RU 486: dose response relationship. *Journal of Clinical Endocrinology and Metabolism* 60: 1–4.

Herrmann W, Wyss R, Riondel A et al (1982) Effet d'un stéroide anti-progéstérone chez la femme: interruption du cycle menstruel et de la grossesse au début. *Comptes Rendus de l'Académie des Sciences, Paris* 294: 933–938.

Herrmann WL, Schindler AM, Wyss R & Bishof P (1985) Effects of the antiprogesterone RU 486 in early pregnancy and during the menstrual cycle. In Baulieu EE & Segal SJ (eds) *The Antiprogestin Steroid RU 486 and Human Fertility Control*, pp 179–198. New York: Plenum Press.

Kovacs L (1985) Termination of very early pregnancy with different doses of RU 486: a phase I controlled clinical trial. In Baulieu EE & Segal SJ (Eds) *The Antiprogestin Steroid RU 486 and Human Fertility Control*, pp 221–234. New York: Plenum Press.

Kovacs L, Sas M, Resch BA et al (1984) Termination of very early pregnancy by RU 486–an antiprogestational compound. *Contraception* **29:** 399–410.

Mishell DR Jr, Shoupe D, Brenner PF et al (1987) Termination of early gestation with the anti-progestin steroid RU 486: medium versus low dose. *Contraception* **35:** 307–321.

Rabe T, Kiesel L, Kellermann J, Weidenhammer K, Runnebaum B & Potts GO (1983) Inhibition of human placental progesterone synthesis and aromatase activity by synthetic steroidogenic inhibitors in vitro. *Fertility and Sterility* **39:** 829–835.

Rådestad A, Christensen NJ & Strömberg L (1988) Cervical ripening with RU 486 in first trimester abortion. A double-blind randomized biomechanical study. *Contraception* (in press).

Rodger MW & Baird DT (1987) Induction of therapeutic abortion in early pregnancy with mifepristone in combination with prostaglandin pessary. *Lancet* **ii:** 1415–1418.

Shoupe D, Mishell DR Jr, Brenner PF & Spitz IM (1986) Pregnancy termination with a high and medium dosage regimen of RU 486. *Contraception* **33:** 455–461.

Smith SK & Kelly RW (1987) The effect of the antiprogestins RU 486 and ZK 98.734 on the synthesis and metabolism of prostaglandin $F_{2\alpha}$ and $E_2$ in separated cells from early human decidua. *Journal of Clinical Endocrinology and Metabolism* **65:** 527–534.

Swahn ML & Bygdeman M (1987) Interruption of early gestation with prostaglandins and antiprogestin. In Diczfalusy E & Bygdeman M (eds) *Fertility Regulation Today and Tomorrow*, Serono Symposia Publications. vol. 36, pp 109–118. New York: Raven Press.

Swahn ML & Bygdeman M (1988) The effect of the antiprogestin RU 486 on uterine contractility and sensitivity to prostaglandin and oxytocin. *British Journal of Obstetrics and Gynaecology* **95:** 126–134.

Swahn ML, Ugocsai G, Bygdeman M, Kovacs L, Belsey EM & Van Look PFA (1988) Effect of oral prostaglandin $E_2$ on uterine contractility and treatment outcome in women receiving RU 486 (mifepristone) for termination of early pregnancy. *Human Reproduction* (submitted for publication).

Ulmann A (1987) Uses of RU 486 for contragestion: an update. *Contraception* **36(Supplement):** 27–31.

Urquhart DR & Templeton AA (1987) Mifepristone (RU 486) and second trimester termination. *Lancet* **ii:** 1405.

Van Look PFA (1988) Antiprogestins: a new era in hormonal fertility regulation. In *Proceedings of the First Congress of the International Society of Gynecological Endocrinology*. Carnforth: Parthenon Publishing.

Vervest HAM & Haspels AA (1985) Preliminary results with the antiprogestational compound RU 486 (mifepristone) for interruption of early pregnancy. *Fertility and Sterility* **44:** 627–632.

Webster MA, Phipps SL & Gillmer MDG (1985) Interruption of first trimester human pregnancy following epostane therapy. Effect of prostaglandin $E_2$ pessaries. *British Journal of Obstetrics and Gynaecology* **92:** 963–968.

WHO Task Force on Postovulatory Methods for Fertility Regulation (1987) Menstrual regulation by intramuscular injection of 16-phenoxy-tetranor $PGE_2$ methyl sulfonylamide or vacuum aspiration. *British Journal of Obstetrics and Gynaecology* **94:** 949–956.

Wiechert R & Neef G (1987) Synthesis of antiprogestational steroids. *Journal of Steroid Biochemistry* **27:** 851–858.

# 8

## Anti-progesterones in obstetrics, ectopic pregnancies and gynaecological malignancy

A. ULMANN
C. DUBOIS

Mifepristone (RU486; Roussel-Uclaf, Paris) is the leading example of a progesterone receptor antagonist. Earlier chapters have concentrated on the use of mifepristone as a contragestive agent for the induction of menstruation and for early pregnancy interruption (Baulieu et al, 1987; Dubois et al, 1988). The focus of this chapter is upon potential additional uses for anti-progesterones: in particular, possible roles of progesterone receptor antagonists for cervical priming, uterine evacuation after fetal death in utero, induction of labour at term gestation and ectopic pregnancy. In addition, some data suggest that anti-progesterones may be useful as therapeutic agents in some progesterone receptor-containing tumours.

### OBSTETRICAL INDICATIONS FOR ANTI-PROGESTERONES

#### Intrauterine pregnancy

*Cervical priming*

The changes in the uterine cervix that occur at the end of pregnancy are likely to be related to the withdrawal of progesterone. If this is true, the administration of anti-progesterones to pregnant women may result in cervical ripening at any stage of pregnancy. This cervical action of anti-progesterones may be direct, or indirect through the induction of uterine contractions.

In the first double-blind study investigating the potential for anti-progesterones to ripen the cervix, mifepristone or placebo was administered double-blind at a dose of 200 mg/day for 2 days prior to vacuum aspiration for interruption of pregnancy, in pregnancies up to 12 weeks of amenorrhoea. The status of the cervix was determined before and after treatment and immediately before vacuum aspiration. Compared with placebo, mifepristone treatment resulted in a significant increase in cervical diameter (6.4 versus 4.3 mm in mifepristone and placebo groups respectively, $p <$

$10^{-4}$; Ulmann and Dubois, unpublished data). In addition, in the mifepristone-treated group, vacuum aspiration was considered significantly easier although operative bleeding was similar in both groups of patients.

In a second study (Lefebvre et al, 1987), mifepristone was given randomly as a single dose at doses between 50 and 600 mg 48 hours prior to vacuum aspiration for interruption of pregnancies up to 12 weeks gestation. Additional patients received placebo treatment. Cervical dilation was measured before and 24 and 48 hours after treatment. A significant increase in cervical dilation was demonstrated 48 hours after treatment at a dose of 100 mg mifepristone. In this dose-finding study, no further dose-dependent increase in cervical dilation occurred at doses of the anti-progesterone above 100 mg. The cervical effect was greater in multiparous women and for those pregnancies greater than 10 weeks' gestation.

In both these studies, tolerance for the anti-progesterone was high and cervical dilation occurred typically without significant pain. The subsequent surgical procedures were facilitated by the cervical dilation and there appeared to be no increase in intraoperative bleeding. When compared with cervical priming with prostaglandins, anti-progesterones appear to result in slower cervical dilation of a smaller magnitude. This effect must be balanced against the absence of pain and the gastrointestinal side-effects which commonly occur with prostaglandin therapy (Bygdeman et al, 1980).

### Anti-progesterones for management of fetal death in utero

Management of fetal death in utero can be a difficult obstetric problem. Typically, the placenta continues to secrete progesterone for days and even weeks after fetal death. For this reason, spontaneous labour may not occur and, in the absence of spontaneous cervical ripening, the induction of labour in a distraught patient can be difficult.

In a pilot study (Cabrol et al, 1985), mifepristone was administered at a dose of 200 mg 12-hourly for 2 days to patients with fetal death in utero for the purpose of blocking progesterone action and inducing labour. Initiation of labour and delivery of the dead fetus and placenta occurred in 8 out of 10 patients. By contrast, administration of mifepristone for second-trimester termination of pregnancy with a living fetus resulted in delivery in only 2 out of 9 subjects. These results suggest that the efficacy of anti-progesterones for the induction of labour in the second and third trimester of pregnancy may be less in the presence of a live fetus but whether this is due to increased progesterone secretion in such pregnancies is unknown.

The efficacy of mifepristone for expulsion of fetal death in utero has now been confirmed through a large-scale double-blind trial involving 92 patients comparing mifepristone (200 mg t.d.s. for 2 days) with placebo (Table 1). Complete expulsion of the fetus and placental contents from the uterus occurred within 72 hours in 29/46 women (63%) after mifepristone but in only 8/46 (17%) after placebo ($p < 0.001$). This effect was independent of the age of gestation and also independent of the interval between fetal death and the administration of the anti-progesterones.

In a related study, Urquart and Templeton (1987) administered mifepristone 200 mg to 40 patients with viable pregnancies between 16 and 18 weeks' gestation. The administration of the anti-progesterone was followed 24 hours later by extra-amniotic infusion of prostaglandin $E_2$ to 20 subjects in this series, whereas the other 20 patients received the prostaglandin infusion only. In the mifepristone group, the induction-to-abortion interval was significantly reduced (mean 9.2 h versus 12.2 h in the absence of mifepristone, $p < 0.005$) and the total dose of prostaglandin required for uterine evacuation was also significantly reduced (11 mg in the mifepristone group versus 18 mg in the control group, $p < 0.001$). This study confirms data from the first trimester of pregnancy (see Chapter 7) indicating that administration of an anti-progesterone will substantially decrease the total amount of exogenous prostaglandin necessary for second-trimester termination of pregnancy.

Table 1. Double-blind study of the efficacy of mifepristone (200 mg t.d.s. for 2 days) for expulsion of a dead fetus.

| | Mifepristone (n = 46) | Placebo (n = 46) | $p$ |
|---|---|---|---|
| Maternal age (year ± s.e.m.) | 27.8 ± 0.8 | 28.9 ± 0.9 | NS |
| Pregnancy age— number of women at the first/second/third trimester | 1/16/27 | 0/16/29 | NS |
| Time elapsed between fetal death and treatment (days ± s.e.m.) | 18.2 ± 4.1 | 15.1 ± 2.5 | NS |
| Number (and %) of women in whom expulsion took place ≤ 72 h after treatment | 29 (63.0) | 8 (17.4) | < 0.001 |

NS = not significant.

*Induction of labour at term gestation*

Anti-progesterones may also be used at the end of pregnancy for induction of labour where this is obstetrically indicated. To date, no clinical trials examining the value of anti-progesterones for termination of pregnancy at term gestation have been reported. Two studies have recently been completed in non-human primates which do address this potential usefulness of progesterone receptor antagonists. The first study was undertaken in 51 term-pregnant cynomolgous monkeys (Wolf et al, 1988a). On day 160 or 161 of gestation (term gestation 167 days) the animals were randomly distributed into four groups. Group A was the control group, group B received mifepristone only (25 mg early in the evening), group C received oxytocin only (20 u intravenously in the morning) while group D received mifepristone followed 12 hours later by oxytocin infusion.

Examination for cervical dilatation and the induction of labour was performed by manual palpation 12 hours after treatment and was repeated if delivery had not occurred within 24 hours. When oxytocin was given alone or with mifepristone, pelvic examinations were made within 15 minutes and hourly until delivery. Mifepristone was effective in promoting cervical dilatation by a simultaneous shortening and softening of the cervix. However, although mifepristone increased uterine contractility, it failed to induce symmetrical and co-ordinated uterine contractions sufficient to induce labour by itself. Oxytocin alone was also ineffective in these non-human primates.

In group D monkeys, the combination of mifepristone and oxytocin resulted in vaginal delivery within 24 hours in 12 out of 14 monkeys. In this group, delivery occurred at $162.5 \pm 1.5$ days of gestation, significantly before the control group (group A: $167.3 \pm 2.4$ days, $p < 0.05$). Amongst all groups, 48 of 49 fetuses delivered alive were thriving at 6 weeks of age. One 3-week-old infant from group D died of unknown causes and there were 2 stillbirths (one in group A, one in group B). In addition, administration of mifepristone appeared to accelerate lactation and increase milk flow, resulting in transiently greater growth rates for babies nursed by mifepristone-treated mothers.

In another set of studies (Wolf et al, 1988), the pharmacokinetics of anti-progesterone administration in both the maternal and fetal compartments were investigated. Monkeys received mifepristone (25 mg in 1 ml ethanol as an intravenous bolus) either at 100–130 days of gestation (group A: $110 \pm 10.3$ days) or at 130–160 days (group B: $139 \pm 8.5$ days). Blood was sampled from the maternal and fetal placental compartments at 5, 15, 30, 60 and 120 minutes for the measurement not only of mifepristone but also its cross-reacting metabolites (N-didemethyl mifepristone, N-monodemethyl mifepristone and propargyl alcohol mifepristone). Plasma concentrations of mifepristone in the maternal circulation did not differ at any time between group A and group B animals. Mifepristone appeared to be immediately transferred into the fetal–placental compartment, reaching a gradient equilibrium within 5 minutes. Concentrations of the anti-progesterone in both mothers and fetuses demonstrated similar distribution and elimination curves. The ratio of the areas beneath the disappearance curves (fetal–placental–maternal) shifted significantly ($p < 0.01$) from 31.2% in second-trimester pregnancies to 17.8% in third-trimester pregnancies. This result may be due to the increased volume of the fetal–placental compartment in the third trimester. Alternatively, this result may arise because the third-trimester placenta is less facilitatory to passage of an anti-progesterone from the maternal compartment.

In human beings (Frydman et al, 1985) as in non-human primates anti-progesterones appear to cross the placenta. There are currently no data indicating the possible usefulness of anti-progesterones for the induction of labour in humans at term gestation. In particular, there are no safety data to demonstrate the absence of any deleterious effects of anti-progesterones in the newborn.


**Ectopic pregnancy**

Ectopic pregnancy has traditionally been managed surgically. In recent years, stimulated by the diagnosis of ectopic pregnancy at an earlier gestation, several groups have reported alternatives to laparotomy for this pregnancy complication. Surgical alternatives include laparoscopic removal of ectopic pregnancy or the aspiration of an ectopic pregnancy using vaginal ultrasound-guided aspirating needles. Medical alternatives to laparotomy for ectopic pregnancy have included the systemic administration of anti-proliferative drugs such as methotrexate. In this setting, the administration of an anti-progesterone may result in the safe disruption of an early ectopic pregnancy and tubal abortion through the fimbrial end of the uterine tube or resorption of the ectopic gestation as a result.

In a preliminary open study (Paris et al, 1984), 8 women with an ectopic pregnancy proven at laparoscopy received 200 mg/day of mifepristone for 4 days. In 7 cases, clinical symptoms disappeared within 24 hours after initiation of treatment and ultrasonography showed a double-layer appearance of the uterine tube, suggesting cleavage between the tubal wall and the pregnancy. A second laparoscopy was performed at day 8 in 7 subjects in this series. In one patient, the haematosalpinx had disappeared and in 4 additional cases it had decreased in size, enabling laparoscopic tubal incision and the expulsion of a clot, without haemorrhage, through the tube in 3 of these 4 patients. In the other 3 women who underwent a second laparoscopy, the haematosalpinx had increased in size and was treated at laparoscopy. In the eighth patient, in whom the ectopic pregnancy was tiny at first laparoscopy, complete clinical regression was obtained and a second laparoscopy was not performed. Interestingly, 2 of these 8 patients subsequently had a normal intrauterine pregnancy. Although this preliminary series appears promising, it does lack a control group; this is especially relevant as spontaneous resolution and cure of ectopic pregnancy have been reported (Garcia et al, 1987).

In the French trials for voluntary interruption of pregnancy with anti-progesterones, 4 of approximately 1000 women treated with mifepristone had a previously undiagnosed ectopic pregnancy. Ectopic pregnancy in these women was diagnosed at the time of final assessment of the efficacy of the anti-progesterone and was discovered in patients classified as failures of mifepristone treatment. These patients subsequently underwent successful routine surgical treatment. It is not possible to exclude the possibility that some additional women with an undiagnosed ectopic pregnancy had successful interruption of the tubal gestation by an anti-progesterone. Nevertheless, the rate of ectopic pregnancy observed in the French trials falls within the reported range of approximately 5 per 1000 conceptions (Meirich, 1981; Westrom et al, 1981) and the efficacy of the anti-progesterone in terminating ectopic pregnancy is still unclear. At the present time, the role of anti-progesterones in the medical treatment of ectopic pregnancy is uncertain.

## PROGESTERONE RECEPTOR-CONTAINING TUMOURS

Progesterone-dependent tumour growth has been demonstrated for various gynaecological malignancies, including those of the breast, endometrium and ovary. Anti-progesterones potentially may inhibit growth of tumours in those organs which do contain progesterone receptors. Some preliminary studies have indicated that further evaluation of the effect of anti-progesterones upon the natural history of some gynaecological malignancies would be worthwhile.

Studies performed in a cultured human breast cancer (NCF7) showed that mifepristone inhibited the growth of these breast cancer cells via the progesterone receptor (Bardon et al, 1985). On the basis of these in vitro results, an open trial was conducted in 27 menopausal or castrated women with advanced breast cancer containing progesterone receptors (Romieu et al, 1987). These patients had all become resistant to conventional therapy. They received mifepristone 50 mg q.i.d. for 1–3 months. The anti-progesterone therapy was well tolerated and, in particular, no side-effects attributable to the anti-glucocorticoid actions of mifepristone were reported. In 6 patients, a transient remission was noted, evidenced by a decrease or a plateau in the circulating concentration of carcinoembryonic antigen. Clearly, these results must be viewed as preliminary and a systematic assessment of the effect of anti-progesterone alone or in combination with anti-oestrogen therapy must be undertaken in breast cancer. Similarly, the possible usefulness of anti-progesterones in other tumours containing progesterone receptors (endometrial cancer, ovarian cancer, meningioma) deserves clinical trials.

## SUMMARY

Table 2 summarizes the proven and potential uses of anti-progesterones in

**Table 2**. Proven and potential uses of anti-progesterones in obstetrics and gynaecology.

| |
|---|
| *Proven uses* |
| Induction of menstruation |
| First- and second-trimester pregnancy termination (in combination with prostaglandins) |
| Cervical ripening |
| Expulsion of a dead fetus in utero |
| |
| *Potential uses* |
| Medical management of ectopic pregnancy |
| Labour induction (in combination with oxytocin) |
| Initiation of lactation |
| Breast cancer, endometrial cancer and other malignancies containing progesterone receptors |

obstetrics and gynaecology. In addition to their role in the induction of menstruation and the interruption of first-trimester pregnancy, anti-progesterones can definitely accelerate cervical ripening and promote the termination of second-trimester pregnancy, especially in combination with exogenous prostaglandins. Furthermore, anti-progesterones can also initiate labour in the obstetric complication of fetal death in utero, leading to delivery of the fetus and placenta without additional medical treatment and without surgery in the majority of patients.

The wider use of anti-progesterones for the induction of labour, with or without other adjuvants such as oxytocin or prostaglandin analogues, is still uncertain and awaits further study. Anti-progesterones may also be useful in the medical treatment of early ectopic pregnancy, either alone or in combination with other medicines. Preliminary results indicate that progesterone receptor antagonists may also be useful both for the initiation and promotion of lactation as well as the possible management of advanced breast cancer containing progesterone receptors. Finally, the usefulness of anti-progesterones in other gynaecological malignancies containing progesterone receptors, such as endometrial or ovarian cancers, awaits further study.

## REFERENCES

Bardon S, Vignon F, Chalbos D & Rochefort M (1985) RU 486, a progestin and glucocorticoid antagonist, inhibits the growth of breast cancer cells via the progesterone receptor. *Journal of Clinical Endocrinology and Metabolism* **50:** 692–697.

Baulieu EE, Ulmann A & Philibert D (1987) Contragestion by antiprogestin RU 486: a review. *Archives of Gynaecology and Obstetrics* **241:** 73–85.

Bygdeman M, Dremme K, Christensen N, Lundstrom V & Green K (1980) A comparison of two stable prostaglandin E analogues for termination of early pregnancy and for cervical dilation. *Contraception* **22:** 471–489.

Cabrol D, Bouvier d'Yvoire M, Mermet E, Cedard L, Sureau C & Baulieu EE (1985) Induction of labour with mifepristone after intrauterine foetal death. *Lancet* **ii:** 1019.

Dubois C, Ulmann A, Aubeny E et al (1988) Contragestion par le RU 486: intérêt de l'association à un dérivé prostaglandine. *Comptes Rendus de l'Académie de Sciences de Paris* **3056:** 57–61.

Frydman R, Taylor S & Ulmann A (1985) Transplacental passage of mifepristone. *Lancet* **ii:** 1252.

Garcia AJ, Aubert JM, Sama J & Josimovich JB (1987) Expectant management of presumed ectopic pregnancy. *Fertility and Sterility* **48:** 395–400.

Lefebevre Y, Proulx L, Cerat Y, Poulin O & Lama E (1987) The effects of mifepristone (RU–38486) on dilation of the cervix in late first trimester abortion. *Abstract to the World Congress on Human Reproduction, Tokyo*

Meirich OK (1981) Ectopic pregnancy during 1961–1978 in Uppsall County, Sweden. Impact of demographic factor on overall incidence. *Acta Obstetrica et Gynecologica Scandinavica* **60:** 545–548.

Paris FX, Henry-Suchet J, Tesquier L, Loysel T, Loffredo V & Pez JM (1984) Le traitement médical des grossesses extra-utérines par le RU 486. *Presse Médicale* **13:** 1219.

Romieu G, Maudelonde T, Ulmann A et al (1987) The antiprogestin RU 486 in advanced breast cancer: preliminary clinical trial. *Bulletin of Cancer* **74:** 455–461.

Urquart DR, Templeton AA (1987) Mifepristone (RU 486) and second-trimester termination. *Lancet* **ii:** 1405.

Westrom L, Bengtsson LP & Mardk PA (1981) Incidence, trends and risks of ectopic pregnancy in a population of women. *British Medical Journal* **282:** 15–18.

Wolf JP, Smosich M, Ulmann A, Baulieu EE & Hodgen GD (1988a) Progesterone antagonist (RU 486) for cervical dilatation labour induction and delivery in monkeys: effectiveness in combination with oxytocin (in press).

Wolf JP, Weyman D, Chillik DF et al (1988b) Transplacental passage of RU 486 antagonist in primates: maternal versus foetal metabolism. *American Journal of Obstetrics and Gynecology* **159:** 238–242.

# 9

# LHRH analogues: their clinical physiology and delivery systems

## H. M. FRASER

### INTRODUCTION

### LHRH: basic research to clinical application

Luteinizing hormone-releasing hormone (LHRH), also known as gonado-trophin-releasing hormone (GnRH), forms an essential link between the central nervous system and the anterior pituitary gland and the control of reproduction. Since its isolation and structural characterization in 1971 a number of model systems have been identified by which the physiological role of LHRH may be studied (Table 1). In turn, some of these approaches have formed the basis for manipulating the LHRH input to the pituitary gonadotrophe both to stimulate, in situations when hypothalamic LHRH is low or absent, or reversibly to inhibit the reproductive system for contraception and for treatment of hormone-dependent disorders. This chapter summarizes the physiological basis for the clinical use of LHRH, the mechanism of action and modes of delivery of its agonist and antagonist analogues and addresses some of the salient issues of control of gonado-trophin release.

That many approaches have been devised to study the physiological role

**Table 1.** Naturally occurring and experimentally induced models for LHRH deprivation.

| Model | Effect |
|---|---|
| *Naturally occurring* | |
| Hypogonadal mouse | Deletion in LHRH gene |
| Kallman's syndrome | Absence of LHRH production |
| Hypothalamic anovulation | Reduced LHRH release |
| Anorexia nervosa | Reduced LHRH release |
| Puberty | Low LHRH release |
| Seasonal breeders | Low LHRH release in non-breeding season |
| *Experimentally induced* | |
| Lesions in arcuate nucleus | Stops LHRH release |
| LHRH antibodies | Prevent LHRH reaching receptor |
| LHRH antagonists | LHRH receptor blockade |
| LHRH agonists | Gonadotrophe 'down-regulation' |

of LHRH stems in part from the fact that attempts to measure the deca-
peptide in the peripheral circulation were confounded by extremely low
concentrations. LHRH is an example of a local hormone travelling between
the blood vessels connecting the hypothalamus and pituitary. Inability to
measure changes in secretion of a hormone in different endocrine states
virtually rules out one of the classic approaches of the endocrinologist in
assessing its physiological role. The fact that LH is released in episodic
pulses was taken as reflecting that a pulse of LHRH drove each of these LH
pulses; most of our information on changes in LHRH output in man is based
on this assumption. The approach of inhibiting the action of LHRH by
neutralization of LHRH by specific antibodies and later by LHRH antagonists helped confirm that each pulse of LH was dependent on LHRH release
from the hypothalamus.

The importance of using pulsatile LHRH in near-physiological regimens
for stimulating pituitary–gonadal function in hypogonadotrophic patients
was not fully appreciated until experiments in the late 1970s by Knobil's
group on monkeys with lesions in the arcuate nucleus to prevent LHRH
release. In this model, LHRH could be replaced at different dose schedules.
Gonadotrophic output and ovulatory cycles could be stimulated by pulses of
exogenous LHRH given at hourly intervals, but not by 3-hourly pulses or
when infused (Knobil, 1980; Pohl et al, 1983). These techniques defined the
physiological role of LHRH and formed the basis for successful treatment of
hypogonadotrophic hypogonadism (Crowley et al, 1985; Wong and Asch,
1987).

When LHRH agonists were evaluated for their ability to induce sustained
gonadotrophin output it was discovered that the initial stimulatory effect
was soon followed by a suppression of pituitary–gonadal function. These
observations were the result of 'down-regulation' by which a cell becomes
refractory to excessive exposure from its trophic hormone—this is now
recognized as a common biological phenomenon. The ability of LHRH
agonists to down-regulate the pituitary gonadotrophe at low doses and
induce a reversible method of gonadal suppression has been widely investigated for the treatment of a wide range of clinical disorders and for contraception during the last ten years.

LHRH antagonists, working by blocking the LHRH receptor, may seem
the more logical choice to suppress pituitary–gonadal function but it has
taken extensive modification of the LHRH molecule to produce compounds
of sufficient potency. Antagonists with clinical potential have only recently
become available. They must still be used in higher doses than the agonists
but have the advantage that they suppress pituitary–ovarian function
immediately, avoiding the stimulatory phase which is obligatory with
agonist administration.

## PHYSIOLOGY OF LHRH

### Synthesis of LHRH

LHRH arises from the post-translational processing of a larger precursor

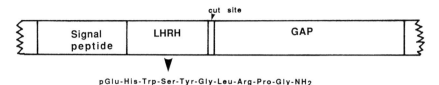

**Figure 1.** Composition of luteinizing hormone-releasing hormone (LHRH) precursor and structure of LHRH. GAP = gonadotrophin-releasing hormone-associated peptide.

molecule (Seeburg and Adelman, 1984; Seeburg et al, 1987). The amino acid sequence of the precursor, derived from the cDNA nucleotide sequence, consists of 92 amino acids. The precursor shows a tripartite structure, consisting of a signal sequence, the LHRH ten amino acid sequence, a site for enzymatic processing, and a 56 amino acid-long peptide which has been termed GnRH-associated peptide (GAP) (Seeburg and Adelman, 1984) (Figure 1). Enzymatic processing produces LHRH, which is identical in all mammalian species, and GAP whose amino acid composition is conserved about 85% between human, rat and mouse. GAP and LHRH have been co-localized within neurones by immunohistochemistry (Ronnekleiv et al, 1987) and expression of the LHRH-GAP gene in rat, mouse and macaque has been demonstrated in cell bodies by in situ hybridization (Standish et al, 1987). LHRH-producing cell bodies are found mainly in the septal preoptic area, diagonal band of Broca, organum vasculosum of the lamina terminalis, and the olfactory bulb.

The hypogonadal mouse is of interest because the LHRH gene is not expressed and these animals lack reproductive function. Exon II, which encodes LHRH and the first 11 residues of GAP, is left intact, but functional LHRH or GAP is not generated because there is a large deletion which has removed the third and fourth exon encoding the 45 C-terminal residues of GAP. Transplantation of normal fetal mouse preoptic tissue into the third ventricle of the hypogonadal mouse results in growth of LHRH fibres from the graft to the host's median eminence, leading to LHRH secretion and stimulation of pituitary–gonadal function (Charlton, 1987). Cure of this trait has been achieved by introduction of intact LHRH gene into the genome of the mutant mice (Mason et al, 1986).

## LHRH and control of LH and follicle-stimulating hormone (FSH) release

There is considerable evidence that LHRH is the sole LH and FSH-releasing hormone (FSH-RH). However the existence of a separate FSH-RH, as predicted from classical endocrinology, cannot be completely ruled out and a number of observations may be taken to question the ability of LHRH to control FSH secretion fully. For example, LHRH is more potent in releasing LH than FSH under most physiological conditions (Yen et al, 1975). It is also clear that removal of the LHRH stimulus has more profound inhibitory effects on LH than on FSH, although this is more apparent in laboratory and veterinary animals than in the primates (Clarke, 1987). FSH secretion can

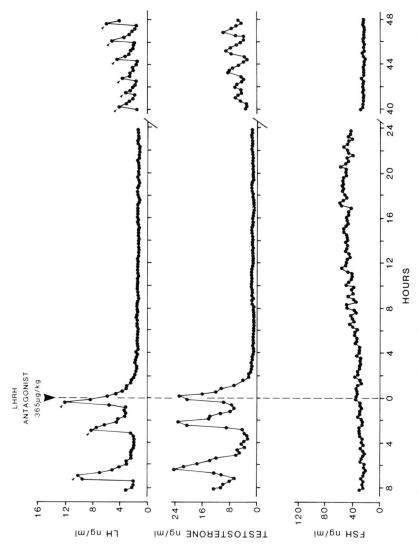

**Figure 2.** Changes in the concentrations of LH, testosterone and FSH in the blood plasma of a Soay ram before and after injection of an LHRH antagonist. Significant LH pulses are indicated by arrows. From Lincoln and Fraser (1987).

remain for some time after withdrawal of LHRH and can persist for several days from pituitaries in vitro. The dependence of LH pulses on LHRH secretion from the hypothalamus is illustrated in Figure 2, which depicts how when a ram was injected with an LHRH antagonist, LH secretion fell immediately while that of FSH persisted (Lincoln and Fraser, 1987). Longer-term suppression of LHRH will suppress FSH output (Fraser, 1986) and it may be that some of the immunoreactive FSH released after administration of LHRH antagonist has reduced biological activity (Dahl et al, 1986; Kessel et al, 1988).

Some studies on purification of hypothalamic extracts have lent support to the idea of a separate FSH-RH (McCann et al, 1986), but after nearly two decades of effort such a factor has yet to be chemically identified.

It has been hypothesized that while LHRH stimulates both synthesis and secretion of LH the secretion of FSH is essentially passive (Clarke, 1987). An additional important factor in control of FSH is that it is much more influenced by the negative feedback effects of the gonadal steroids and inhibin at the level of the pituitary than is LH. Reduction in LHRH stimulation is associated with reduction in gonadal steroids and inhibin, so removal of this negative influence could contribute to the maintained FSH secretion.

Since modulation of release of the two gonadotrophins can occur by influence of gonadal steroids and inhibin at the level of the gonadotrophe to suppress FSH secretion, it is generally believed that LHRH is the GnRH. Perhaps the most convincing evidence we have for LHRH controlling both hormones is that pulsatile administration of LHRH in LHRH deficiency results in expression of full pituitary–gonadal function (Knobil, 1980; Crowley et al, 1985).

## Other peptides involved in control of LH and FSH release

During the last few years, a number of neuropeptides have been suggested as acting as modulators of LHRH action at the pituitary level or acting independently on the gonadotrophe. These peptides have been evaluated using pituitary culture systems but evidence for in vivo confirmation of these effects is generally lacking. For example, GAP has recently been detected in hypophyseal portal blood and may be co-released with LHRH (Clarke et al, 1987a). The demonstration that GAP, obtained by engineering a bacterial expression vector for microbial GAP synthesis, stimulated the release of gonadotrophins from rat pituitary cells—although with lower potency than LHRH—and inhibited release of prolactin led to much speculation on a possible physiological role (Nikolics et al, 1985). Since the true nature of hypothalamic control of prolactin release has still to be elucidated, the concept of a concomitant release of LHRH and GAP causing an inverse relationship between gonadotrophin release and prolactin secretions has some attractions, but most observations of physiological condition do not support this idea.

There is reason to believe that GAP may be further broken down into smaller fragments. When tested in human and baboon pituitary cultures,

GAP 14-26 and 14-36 stimulated LH release, but high concentrations were required (Millar et al, 1986; Milton et al, 1987). The question of whether this action is mediated via the LHRH receptor initially suggested an independent site (Millar et al, 1986) but subsequent studies showed that GAP 14-36 displaced labelled LHRH from its receptor and that its action was prevented by LHRH antagonist, suggesting it was acting via the same binding site (Milton et al, 1987).

There has been concern that the biological activity of some GAP preparations may be the result of contamination with LHRH or its agonists during column purification. Several other groups using synthetic GAP in a number of in vitro systems have failed to demonstrate any effect on prolactin or the gonadotrophins (see discussion after Seeburg et al, 1987). These problems, together with the large amounts required for biological effects, currently cast doubt on the physiological significance of the gonadotrophin-releasing properties of GAP.

The recent sequencing of ovarian inhibin will allow the evaluation of its putative role in selective suppression of FSH secretion as well as its function as an intragonadal regulator (McLachlan et al, 1987). Inhibin is a glycoprotein consisting of two disulphide-linked subunits. Surprisingly, it has been reported that two proteins derived from the smaller ($\beta$) subunit stimulate FSH release, but not LH release, from rat pituitary cells in vitro (Ling et al, 1986; Vale et al, 1986). These subunits have been termed activin and FSH-releasing peptide (FRP). During coincubation, inhibin bioactivity predominated. It will be of particular interest to determine whether the hypothalamus secretes these peptides, although their specificity and their action in vivo have yet to be established.

## LHRH secretion and control of the menstrual cycle

As described above, difficulties in measurement of LHRH in the portal blood have proved an obstacle in understanding its physiological control. Surgery and anaesthetics reduced hypothalamic activity, compromising LHRH release but after many years skilful techniques were devised which allowed collection of portal blood in conscious animals. These experiments confirmed the pulsatile nature of LHRH secretion and that LHRH pulses preceded LH pulses (Clarke, 1987; Clarke et al, 1987b; Caraty and Locatelli, 1988) and indicate that pulse frequency is highest after removal of gonadal steroids.

Detailed evaluation of LHRH secretion at different stages of the menstrual cycle has not been possible in primates and changes in LHRH pulse frequency are considered to be reflected by changes in LH pulse frequency. The half-life of LH is between 30 and 50 min and since pulses can occur at intervals of 1 h, the frequency of collection of blood samples has had to be every 10–15 min or less to detect changes in pulse frequency reliably. Several detailed evaluations of changes in LH pulse frequency throughout the menstrual cycle and in anovular conditions have been described (reviewed by Crowley et al, 1985). However, while the frequency and amplitude of the LHRH signal is governed by the feedback of the gonadal steroids, this message is also modulated at the level of the pituitary gonadotrophe by the gonadal steroids and inhibin to vary the amplitude of the LH and FSH pulses and their ratio (Yen et al, 1975).

During the early follicular phase, LH pulses occur at a frequency of approximately 90 min but are almost suspended during sleep. By the mid follicular phase the frequency of LH pulses increases to every 60 min, amplitude decreases and pulses begin to be retained during sleep. Up to this stage of the cycle, blockade of LHRH by LHRH antagonist for 3 days causes suppression of LH and FSH secretion and a subsequent fall in serum oestradiol, reflecting the atresia of the selected follicle; then the whole process must be re-initiated (Kenigsberg and Hodgen, 1986; Mais et al, 1986; Fraser, 1987).

By the late follicular phase LH pulse frequency is increased further. The negative feedback effects of the rising concentrations of oestradiol, which has a selectivity for suppression of FSH, change to a positive feedback and the resultant LH (and FSH) surge is composed of rapid-frequency high-amplitude LH pulses. The LHRH signal is amplified by increasing pituitary responsiveness to LHRH (Yen et al, 1975) and increased numbers of LHRH receptors (Adams and Spies, 1981) which are brought about by the pattern of LHRH release and by direct action of oestradiol on the pituitary. An increase in LHRH output from the hypothalamus has been demonstrated by studies in the rhesus monkey (Levine et al, 1985), although it is of modest magnitude and duration compared to the LH surge, giving further support to the concept that the raised pituitary responsiveness is an important part of the mechanism (Knobil, 1980). Indeed we find this period relatively resistant to the inhibitory effects of LHRH antagonist (Fraser, 1987). After ovulation, with the secretion of progesterone, there is a slowing of LH pulse frequency and increased amplitude. This pattern becomes more pronounced as the luteal phase progresses (Crowley et al, 1985) and is the result of a negative feedback effect of progesterone at the level of the hypothalamus (Yen et al, 1975; Ferin et al, 1984).

In patients with hypothalamic amenorrhoea, LHRH secretion may be absent, slowed down or intermittent (Crowley et al, 1985). The essential requirement for treatment is that exogenous LHRH is administered in a pulsatile mode at a frequency of every 1–2 h (Wong and Asch, 1987). This does not mimic completely the true physiological situation, but is sufficiently close to leave the pituitary to translate the uniform LHRH profile and create normal profiles of LH and FSH; restore follicular development; cause an LH surge; induce ovulation and maintain successful luteal function.

## Mechanism of action of LHRH

The action of LHRH is transmitted via binding to receptors localized on the plasma membrane of pituitary gonadotrophes which then generate intra-cellular messengers. The number of these receptors is influenced by the pattern of LHRH exposure, being reduced in number when exposure to LHRH is removed by LHRH antibodies and up-regulated by pulses of LHRH in hypogonadal mice (Fraser, 1986; Sandow, 1983; Clayton, 1987). These changes may contribute to changes in gonadotrophe responsiveness.

As with other peptides, there are large numbers of 'spare' receptors on the pituitary gonadotrophe so modulation of receptor numbers is likely to be of less physiological importance than alteration of post-receptor mechanisms.

Since LH release is detected within 1–2 min of LHRH administration, these post-receptor changes must occur extremely rapidly and must also have longer-acting consequences to increase gonadotrophin biosynthesis. As with other peptide hormones, these actions are mediated via second messenger systems; the most important for LHRH action involves the breakdown of polyphosphoinositides to generate diacylglycerol and inositol triphosphate (Clayton, 1987; Conn et al, 1987). These messengers activate the phosphorylating enzyme protein kinase C and calcium mobilization respectively. LHRH also stimulates synthesis of LH and FSH, which are composed of a common $\alpha$ subunit and a $\beta$ subunit which renders specificity. These subunits are encoded by single genes which are separately regulated. Further investigation of these intracellular mechanisms are required to elucidate the interplay between LHRH and the gonadal steroids and inhibin in control of LH and FSH synthesis and release.

## MANIPULATION OF GONADOTROPHE FUNCTION BY LHRH ANALOGUES

### LHRH agonists

LHRH agonists were conceived by identifying the sites of enzymatic degradation of LHRH and modifying these positions to increase resistance to peptidases and to enhance affinity of receptor binding. The chemists found development of highly active compounds relatively straightforward by substitution of a bulky hydrophobic D amino acid in position 6. In several compounds the C-terminal glycinamide residue is replaced by an ethylamide group, which has an additive effect (Table 2; Conn et al, 1987; Vickery and Nestor, 1987). The agonists are 50–200 times more potent than LHRH in releasing gonadotrophins. However, their main application since their introduction some ten years ago has been to suppress gonadotrophe function by chronic exposure. In general, the biological properties of all agonists are the same and those of lower potency need simply be used in higher doses.

**Table 2.** Structures of some LHRH agonists.

| Structure | Name | Company |
|---|---|---|
| [D-Trp$^6$] LHRH | Tryptorelin | Debiopharm |
| [D-Nal(2)$^6$] LHRH | Nafarelin | Syntex |
| [D-Trp$^6$,Pro$^9$Net] 1-9 LHRH | – | Salk Institute |
| [D-Trp$^6$,NMeLeu$^7$,Pro$^9$Net] 1-9 LHRH | Lutrelin | Wyeth |
| [D-Leu$^6$,Pro$^9$Net] 1-9 LHRH | Leuprolide | Abbott |
| [D-His(Bzl)$^6$,Pro$^9$Net] 1-9 LHRH | Histerelin | Ortho |
| [D-Ser(But)$^6$,Pro$^9$Net] 1-9 LHRH | Buserelin | Hoechst |
| [D-Ser(But)$^6$,AzaGly$^{10}$] LHRH | Zoladex | ICI |

## Down-regulation by LHRH agonists

Chronic exposure of the pituitary gonadotrophes to LHRH agonists leads to suppression of pituitary–gonadal function by complex mechanisms. The most important are:

1. The over-riding of pulsatile gonadotrophin release;
2. Desensitization of the gonadotrophe, particularly at the post-receptor level;
3. Inducing production of altered forms of gonadotrophin with reduced biological activity.

Initial exposure to LHRH agonist is characterized by marked elevations in serum gonadotrophin concentrations lasting several hours. However, continued administration is associated with decreased pituitary responsiveness which will eventually lead to disruption and suppression of the pituitary–ovarian axis. This effect is dependent on the dose and potency of the agonist and the time and frequency of administration. Once-daily administration produces a daily episode of gonadotrophin secretion which becomes less as the treatment is continued. Continued exposure induced by infusion or by a depot formulation is associated with the initial stimulatory phase only and is more suppressive than once-daily administration.

## Delivery systems for LHRH agonists and endocrine effects

The fact that LHRH agonists are inactivated orally meant that alternative routes of delivery had to be investigated (Table 3). While pilot studies may be performed using daily injections, the development of nasal spray delivery systems allowed widespread studies on the clinical and contraceptive use of the agonists. The efficacy is much lower than compared with injection, being 3–5% for buserelin and 10% for nafarelin (Sandow et al, 1986, 1987; Vickery and Nestor, 1987). However, acceptance is good and many large-scale clinical trials have been performed using nasal sprays.

Daily low-dose agonist administration by nasal spray may be associated with either intermittent periods of oestradiol secretion indicative of follicular maturation or more complete ovarian suppression. In both situations ovulation does not occur since the ability to induce an LH surge is impaired (Fraser, 1981; Bergquist et al, 1982). The follicular development probably results from agonist-induced gonadotrophin release together with incom-

Table 3. Examples of modes of administration of LHRH agonists in clinical use.

| Mode | Availability | Frequency | Dose |
|------|-------------|-----------|------|
| Subcutaneous injection | All agonists | Daily | 50–500 µg |
| Nasal spray | Buserelin | Daily | 300–1200 µg |
|  | Nafarelin |  | 125–600 µg |
| Depots |  |  |  |
| Polymer implant | Zoladex | Monthly | 3.6 mg |
|  | Buserelin | 3-monthly | 3–6 mg |
| Microspheres | Tryptorelin | Monthly | 3 mg |

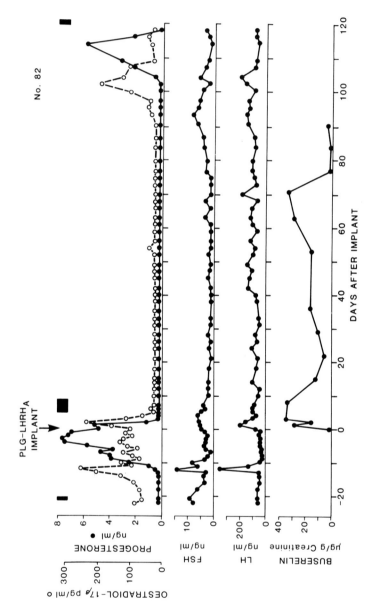

**Figure 3.** Serum concentrations of LH, FSH, oestradiol and progesterone and urinary excretion of buserelin in a stumptailed macaque implanted subcutaneously with buserelin in a PLG matrix. ■ = Menstrual bleeding. From Fraser et al (1987b).

pletely suppressed basal gonadotrophin secretion. It had been hoped that continued low-dose LHRH agonist administration could be developed for contraception but the individual variation in response in relation to oestrogen production during long-term use has proved a major obstacle (Fraser and Baird, 1987). With daily administration of higher doses of agonist by nasal spray, the pituitary can still respond to the agonist—albeit at a reduced rate—and it is likely that between doses the normal pulsatile LH secretion is suppressed because of the reduced responsiveness to endogenous LHRH (Hardt and Schmidt-Gollwitzer, 1984).

With continuous infusion of LHRH agonist the events are more pronounced and there is less individual variation. Pituitary gonadotrophin content and numbers of LHRH receptors are reduced in rats and in sheep more markedly than by daily administration (Sandow, 1983). Gonadotrophin levels are soon suppressed and LH secretion becomes non-pulsatile (Figures 3 and 4) (Healy et al, 1986; Fraser et al, 1987b).

Considerable emphasis has been placed on the development of slow-release formulations, either as microcapsules by intramuscular or subcutaneous injections, or as small rods or discs injected subcutaneously into the anterior abdominal wall. These lead to more effective suppression at a smaller dose, prevent problems of compliance and are generally more

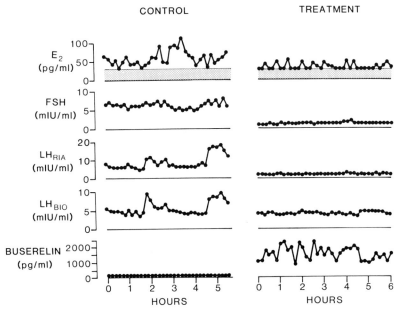

**Figure 4.** Comparison of serum oestradiol ($E_2$), FSH and LH concentrations, as measured by radioimmunoassay (RIA) and bioassay (BIO), in the early follicular phase of the normal menstrual cycle (control) with the same hormones plus buserelin concentrations in a patient after 6 weeks of buserelin infusion. A blood sample was drawn every 10 min for 6 h. The stippled area indicates sensitivity for the serum oestradiol radioimmunoassay. Note the lower oestradiol, FSH and LH concentrations and the abolition of pulsatile LH secretion during buserelin treatment. PLG = polylactide–glycolide copolymer (75 : 25). From Healy et al (1986).

convenient for therapeutic application lasting longer than a month. The most commonly used depot consists of the agonist dispersed in a bio-degradable lactide–glycolide co-polymer, similar in composition to absorbable sutures. According to dose or composition, the duration of release of peptide from these preparations can be adjusted to 1 or 3 months or even longer (Walker et al, 1984; Sandow et al, 1986; Fraser et al, 1987b; Lahlou et al, 1987; West and Baird, 1987; West et al, 1987; Zorn et al, 1988).

Some studies have described a rise in FSH secretion in women after several months of continued agonist treatment by LHRH agonist implant (Walker et al, 1984; West and Baird, 1987; Fraser, unpublished observations). A number of factors may contribute to this surprising phenomenon. The fall in FSH during the first 1–2 weeks of treatment may be due not only to down-regulation by the agonist, but also to the initial rise in gonadal steroids and inhibin causing a negative feedback effect at the pituitary level. Once the gonads become inactive this negative feedback effect is removed and this may precipitate an autonomous release of FSH. It has yet to be determined to what extent the remaining secretion of FSH is due to stimulation by the agonist as well as the degree of the bioactivity of the FSH being measured by radioimmunoassay. The level of FSH does not stimulate follicular development, for which a certain threshold is likely to be required (Zeleznik and Kubik, 1986).

Chronic agonist treatment induces changes in the composition of the LH and FSH molecules being released. When antibodies which cross-react with both normal LH and the α subunit are employed, a decreasing bioactive: immunoactive ratio for LH is observed (Meldrum et al, 1984). This is due in part to an increase in the α subunit concentrations while the β subunit concentrations are decreased (Lahlou et al, 1987). Effects of chronic LHRH agonist treatment on expression of the LH subunit genes have been studied in rats. The levels of β subunit mRNA are unaltered while those of the β subunit are reduced, confirming the dissociation of effects at the pituitary gonadotrophe (Lalloz et al, 1988).

Thus chronic LHRH agonist administration is a very effective way of suppressing ovarian activity. In treatment of oestrogen-dependent disorders, the initial stimulatory phase of agonist is undesirable. When treatment is started in the follicular phase this induces an oestrogen rise which may last 2–3 weeks. This rise tends to be reduced if treatment is started earlier in the cycle: the first 1–2 days of menses are convenient. Beginning treatment during the luteal phase has the advantage of restricting the stimulatory phase of the agonist. On luteal demise the pituitary cannot respond by raising FSH output to stimulate follicular development and no further oestrogen rises occur (Fraser and Sandow, 1985; Healy et al, 1986). However, the patient must ensure that pregnancy does not occur during that cycle.

## Extrapituitary effects of LHRH analogues

The understanding of the mechanism of action of LHRH agonists has been complicated by direct gonadal effects of LHRH and its agonists observed in the rat. Up to 24 h exposure in vivo in hypophysectomized rats or rat gonadal tissue in vitro can lead to increased steroidogenesis while longer-term exposure causes inhibition of gonadotrophin-induced steroidogenesis (Hsueh and Jones, 1981). These effects are mediated via high-affinity receptors for LHRH similar to those found in the pituitary. However, these effects seem to be confined to the rat. There is little convincing evidence for such actions on human or monkey gonadal tissue. Follicular development can be induced by exogenous gonadotrophins in women treated with LHRH agonists and, while some workers have attributed the higher doses of gonadotrophins required to stimulate follicular development in these women to a direct ovarian effect, this may be due rather to the low levels of endogenous LH and FSH. LHRH receptors are not present on human gonadal tissue but low-affinity binding sites are to be found on the human ovary, the placenta and some breast tumours. Despite extensive investigations, the significance of these binding sites remains to be established and it is unlikely that they could be activated by the concentrations of agonist used clinically (Fraser and Eidne, 1988).

## LHRH antagonists

Beginning during the early 1970s a series of increasingly potent antagonists has been synthesized, but effective receptor blockade has been difficult to achieve—the chemists have now produced over 2000 analogues. The development process involved a stepwise introduction of hydrophobic residues which block proteolysis, increase LHRH receptor affinity and prolong the pharmacokinetics of the molecule (Folkers et al, 1987; Vickery and Nestor, 1987). Figure 5 shows examples of the complex unnatural and/or D-amino acids which have been introduced in the LHRH molecule: in current compounds only positions 4 and 9 of LHRH are maintained without change.

pGlu$^1$, His$^2$, Trp$^3$, Ser$^4$, Trp$^5$, Gly$^6$, Leu$^7$, Arg$^8$, Pro$^9$, Gly$^{10}$-NH$_2$      LHRH

[N-Ac-D-Nal(2)$^1$,D-pCl-Phe$^2$,D-Trp$^3$,D-hArg(Et$_2$)$^6$,D-Ala$^{10}$] LHRH      Detirelix (Syntex)

[N-Ac-D-Nal(2)$^1$,D-pCl-Phe$^2$,D-Pal$^3$,Lys(Nic)$^5$,D-Lys(Nic)$^6$,Lys(iPr)$^8$,D-Ala$^{10}$]*      LHRH

**Figure 5.** Structure of LHRH and of two LHRH antagonists.* From Folkers et al (1987).

Potencies have increased by more than one million from the first antagonists in an effort to obtain compounds which can be used effectively in humans in acceptable doses and without side-effects which involve histamine release activated by the complex amino acid formulations (see below). The most recent advances have produced antagonists with gonadotrophin-suppressing action lasting over a week after a single administration in monkeys. This long action seems to be related to the antagonists, which are dissolved in propylene glycol, coming out of solution after injection and forming a depot. These compounds have extremely low histamine-releasing activity and should herald greater advances in clinical studies which have progressed comparatively slowly to date.

Even with potent antagonists, administration of exogenous LHRH can still induce LH release (Weinbauer et al, 1984; Marshall et al, 1986), suggesting that it is difficult to occupy all LHRH receptors; activation of low numbers of receptors can lead to considerable biological action. From studies in the rat it is apparent that LHRH antagonists have little short-term effect on pituitary gonadotrophin content so it may take long-term administration before the pituitary becomes markedly less responsive to LHRH. Perhaps the removal of negative feedback results in increased secretion of endogenous LHRH (Figure 2; Lincoln and Fraser, 1987), which also helps counteract effects of the antagonists.

Antagonists have the advantage of inducing immediate inhibition of LH and FSH release and hence reduction in gonadal activity. Furthermore, they can be used to curtail the menstrual cycle by intermittent administration, thus preventing continued development of the selected follicle when administered during the mid follicular phase (Kenigsberg and Hodgen, 1986; Mais et al, 1986; Fraser, 1987; Kessel et al, 1988). Early reports claimed that administration of quite weak LHRH antagonists during the late follicular phase could prevent the mid-cycle LH surge and ovulation, but in our experience in macaques, this period is relatively resistant to antagonist (Fraser, 1987), probably because of 'fail-safe' mechanisms to induce an LH surge (Knobil, 1980) and because the maturing follicle becomes less dependent on gonadotrophin stimulation (Zeleznik and Kubik, 1986).

During the luteal phase, administration of a LHRH antagonist will induce a reduction in progesterone secretion in response to the fall in serum LH concentrations (Collins et al, 1986; Mais et al, 1986; Fraser et al, 1987). If LH is suppressed for less than 3 days during the early–mid luteal phase, progesterone secretion can usually recover, while longer-term treatment induces luteolysis. Late luteal phase is more susceptible to complete suppression by administration of LHRH antagonist.

The absence of an initial stimulatory effect should make the antagonist of special use when treatment schedules are for the short term, as in ovulation induction by exogenous gonadotrophins. The antagonists may be investigated in disorders which have proved relatively resistant to agonist therapy, such as polycystic ovarian syndrome. However, it seems that satisfactory suppression of pituitary gonadotrophe function can be achieved by down-regulation rather than by receptor blockade, so that it is unlikely that the more complex antagonist compounds will replace agonist implants for long-term therapy.

### Side-effects of LHRH analogues

Side-effects of LHRH and its analogues can be divided into those directly due to the peptides themselves or their delivery systems, and those induced by the changes in the gonadal steroids. LHRH agonist administration by nasal spray is occasionally associated with nasal irritation or a bad taste in the mouth but is otherwise well tolerated. In the case of LHRH agonist deposits, rare local reactions at the site of injection are thought to be due to the carrier material.

A small number of patients treated chronically with LHRH pulses develop urticarial reaction at the injection site which necessitates cessation of therapy. An anaphylactic reaction involving IgE antibodies has been described (MacLeod et al, 1987). Circulating IgG antibodies have been produced in a small number of patients treated for long periods with pulsatile LHRH. These antibodies are sometimes associated with failure of therapy, although antibody titre is frequently very low (Meakin et al, 1985; MacLeod et al, 1987).

LHRH agonists can be classed as 'foreign' peptides because of the presence of their D-amino acid substitutions. However, despite their widespread use no reactions directly attributable to their structure have been reported (Sandow et al, 1986; Vickery and Nestor, 1987). One reason may be because they are effective in such low doses, particularly when administered via slow-release depot formulations.

Certain LHRH antagonists are formed of more complex molecules; since they had to be used at high doses, this caused changes in vascular permeability when they were administered to rats. Transient local erythema, induration and flushing were found in some patients. These side-effects stem from activation of histamine release, a phenomenon associated with peptides having positively charged D-amino acids, in particular with antagonists having a D-Arg in position 6 (Folkers et al, 1987; Vickery and Nestor, 1987). These compounds have now been superseded by antagonists with much reduced side-effects.

The endocrine side-effects of LHRH analogue therapy are related to suppression of oestrogen production and are dependent upon the dose and duration of therapy. Since many recent studies have employed slow-release depot formulations or used agonist for treatment of endometriosis or uterine fibroids, in which removal of oestrogen has been the rationale behind the therapy, marked suppression of oestrogen has been commonly reported. The immediate consequences are hot flushes in almost all patients, while vaginal dryness, decreased libido and headache are reported by a minority of women (Fraser and Baird, 1987; Henzel et al, 1988). The side-effects are, therefore, significant but are generally well tolerated. Comparison with danazol in the treatment of endometriosis shows that the menopausal symptoms induced by the agonist are much more acceptable than the common androgenic side-effects of danazol (Henzel et al, 1988).

It is of greater concern that prolonged use of LHRH agonists may be associated with hypo-oestrogenic bone loss. When this was examined by quantitative computerized tomography of the distal radius, bone density was found to be unchanged after 6–12 months of LHRH agonist treatment (Comite and Jensen, 1988). However, examination of vertebral bone showed a small but significant decrease (Matta et al, 1987). From studies on oestrogen replacement in ovariectomized women and in the preliminary results available from women receiving LHRH agonist it is likely that this bone loss will be recovered on discontinuing treatment (Waibel et al, 1988). It has been suggested that concurrent administration of calcitonin, calcium or fluorides may prevent bone loss. Occasional small rises in oestradiol not easily detectable by assays in general use may be important in maintaining some protection against the unwanted effects of hypo-oestrogenism. Administering doses of agonist which cause less suppression of oestradiol, or even administration of small doses of oestrogen, would be likely to overcome this problem but it must be determined whether this would decrease the efficacy of therapy. Clearly, these complex issues will require investigation in order to determine acceptable duration of therapy.

For a number of conditions such as endometriosis there are various factors, in addition to oestradiol, whose involvement in the disease requires to be resolved. It may be that using LHRH analogues to suppress oestrogen production in combination with compounds using another site of action will lead to more effective therapy. For example, in some patients there is an autoimmune aspect to endometriosis and autoantibodies may contribute to the infertility in these patients, having a disruptive effect on implantation. One of the actions of danazol is to suppress these antibodies (Hill et al, 1987), suggesting that combination of LHRH agonists with agents which limit the effects of the autoantibodies may be more successful in relieving symptoms and increasing pregnancy rates post-treatment.

## SUMMARY

LHRH, produced in the hypothalamus from a precursor molecule, forms an essential link between the central nervous system and the anterior pituitary gland and the control of reproduction. It is secreted in a pulsatile manner and in patients who lack the hormone it is necessary to replace LHRH in a near-physiological mode. Chronic exposure of the pituitary gonadotrophes to LHRH by infusion and to LHRH agonists leads to suppression of pituitary–gonadal function by mechanisms which involve:

1. The over-riding of pulsatile gonadotrophin release;
2. Desensitization of the gonadotrophe, particularly at the post-receptor level;
3. Inducing production of altered forms of gonadotrophin with reduced biological activity.

An effective and reversible suppression of pituitary–ovarian function can be readily obtained by administering LHRH agonists by nasal spray or by slow-release depot formulations lasting 1–3 months. LHRH agonist therapy is without serious side-effects but more work is required to evaluate the role of oestrogen in maintaining bone density. Suppression of the gonadotrophe can also be obtained by the more conventional approach of receptor blockade by LHRH antagonists. These have the advantage of causing immediate pituitary suppression but higher doses are required than for agonists. LHRH antagonists suitable for clinical evaluation have only recently become available.

## REFERENCES

Adams TE & Spies HG (1981) GnRH receptor binding and pituitary responsiveness in estradiol primed monkeys. *Science* 213: 1388–1390.

Bergquist C, Nillius SJ & Wide L (1982) Long-term intranasal luteinizing hormone-releasing hormone agonist treatment for contraception. *Fertility and Sterility* 38: 190–193.

Caraty A & Locatelli A (1988) Effect of time after castration on secretion of LHRH and LH in the ram. *Journal of Reproduction and Fertility* 82: 263–269.

Clarke IJ (1987) New concepts in gonadotropin-releasing hormone action on the pituitary gland. *Seminars in Reproductive Endocrinology* 5: 345–352.

Clarke IJ, Cummins JT, Karsch FJ, Seeburg PH & Nikolics K (1987a) GnRH-associated peptide (GAP) is cosecreted with GnRH into the hypophyseal portal blood of ovariectomized sheep. *Biochemical and Biophysical Research Communications* 143: 665–671.

Clarke IJ, Thomas GB, Yao B & Cummins JT (1987b) GnRH secretion throughout the ovine oestrous cycle. *Neuroendocrinology* 46: 82–88.

Clayton RN (1987) Gonadotrophin releasing hormone: from physiology to pharmacology. *Clinical Endocrinology* 26: 361–384.

Collins RL, Sopelak VM, Williams RF & Hodgen GD (1986) Prevention of gonadotropin-releasing hormone antagonist induced luteal regression by concurrent exogenous pulsatile gonadotropin administration in monkeys. *Fertility and Sterility* 46: 945–953.

Comite F & Jensen P (1988) Bone density changes associated with GnRH analogues. *Gynecological Endocrinology* 2(suppl 1): abstract 095.

Conn PM, Huckle WR, Andrews WV & McArdle CA (1987) The molecular mechanism of action of gonadotropin releasing hormone (GnRH) in the pituitary. *Recent Progress in Hormone Research* 43: 29–67.

Crowley WF, Filicori M, Spratt DI & Santoro NF (1985) The physiology of gonadotrophin-releasing hormone (GnRH) in men and women. *Recent Progress in Hormone Research* 41: 473–525.

Charlton HM (1987) Neural transplants and the repair of neural endocrine and reproductive deficiencies. *Oxford Reviews of Reproductive Biology* 9: 379–397. J. Clarke (ed.).

Dahl KD, Pavlou SN, Kovacs WJ & Hsueh AJW (1986) The changing ratio of serum bioactive to immunoreactive follicle-stimulating hormone in normal men following treatment with a potent gonadotropin releasing hormone antagonist. *Journal of Clinical Endocrinology and Metabolism* 63: 792–794.

Ferin M, Van Vugt D & Wardlaw S (1984) The hypothalamic control of the menstrual cycle and the role of endogenous opioid peptides. *Recent Progress in Hormone Research* 40: 441–485.

Folkers K, Bowers C, Tang PFL et al (1987) Specificity of design to achieve antagonists of LHRH of increasing effectiveness in therapeutic activity. In Vickery BN & Nestor JJ (eds) *LHRH and its Analogs: Contraceptive and Therapeutic Applications*, part 2, pp 25–36. Lancaster: MTP Press.

Fraser HM (1981) Effect of oestrogen on gonadotrophin release in stumptailed monkeys (*Macaca arctoides*) treated chronically with an agonist analogue of LH-RH. *Journal of Endocrinology* 91: 525–530.

Fraser HM (1986) LHRH immunoneutralization: basic studies and prospects for practical application. In Talwar GP (ed.) *Immunological Approaches to Contraception and Promotion of Fertility*, pp 125–141. New York: Plenum Press.

Fraser HM (1987) LHRH antagonists and female reproductive function. In Vickory BH & Nestor JJ (eds) *LHRH and its Analogs: Contraceptive and Therapeutic Applications*, part 2, pp 227–244. Lancaster: MTP Press.

Fraser HM & Baird DT (1987) Clinical applications of LHRH analogues. *Clinical Endocrinology and Metabolism* 1: 43–70.

Fraser HM & Eidne KA (1988) Extra pituitary actions of LHRH analogues and LHRH-like peptides. In Shaw RW & Marshall JC (eds) *LHRH Analogues in Gynaecological Practice*. Bristol: John Wright.

Fraser HM & Sandow J (1985) Suppression of follicular maturation by infusion of a luteinizing hormone releasing hormone agonist starting during the late luteal phase in the stumptailed macaque monkey. *Journal of Clinical Endocrinology and Metabolism* 60: 579–584.

Fraser HM, Nestor JJ & Vickery BH (1987a) Suppression of luteal function by an LHRH antagonist during the early luteal phase in the stumptailed macaque and the effects of subsequent administration of hCG. *Endocrinology* **121:** 612–618.

Fraser HM, Sandow J, Seidel H & von Rechenberg W (1987b) An implant of a gonadotrophin releasing hormone agonist (buserelin) which suppresses ovarian function in the macaque for 3–5 months. *Acta Endocrinologica* **115:** 521–527.

Hardt W & Schmidt-Gollwitzer M (1984) Sustained gonadal suppression in fertile women with the LHRH agonist buserelin. *Clinical Endocrinology* **19:** 613–617.

Healy DL, Lawson SR, Abbott M, Baird DT & Fraser HM (1986) Towards removing uterine fibroids without surgery: subcutaneous infusion of a luteinizing hormone-releasing hormone agonist commencing in the luteal phase. *Journal of Clinical Endocrinology and Metabolism* **63:** 616–625.

Henzel MR, Corson SL, Moghissi KS et al (1988) Administration of nasal nafarelin as compared with oral danazol for endometriosis. *New England Journal of Medicine* **318:** 485–489.

Hill JA, Barbieri RL & Anderson DJ (1987) Immunosuppressive effects of danazol in vitro. *Fertility and Sterility* **48:** 414–418.

Hsueh AJ & Jones PBC (1981) Extrapituitary actions of the gonadotropin-releasing hormone. *Endocrine Reviews* **2:** 437–461.

Kenigsberg D & Hodgen GD (1986) Ovulation inhibition by administration of weekly gonadotropin-releasing hormone antagonist. *Journal of Clinical Endocrinology and Metabolism* **62:** 734–736.

Kessel B, Dahl KD, Kazer RR et al (1988) The dependency of bioactive follicle-stimulating hormone secretion on gonadotropin-releasing hormone in hypogonadal and cycling women. *Journal of Clinical Endocrinology and Metabolism* **66:** 361–366.

Knobil E (1980) The neuroendocrine control of the menstrual cycle. *Recent Progress in Hormone Research* **36:** 53–88.

Lahlou N, Roger M, Chaussain JL et al (1987) Gonadotrophin and α-subunit secretion during long term pituitary suppression by D-Trp6-luteinizing hormone-releasing hormone microcapsules as treatment of precocious puberty. *Journal of Clinical Endocrinology and Metabolism* **65:** 946–953.

Lalloz MRA, Detta A & Clayton RN (1988) Gonadotropin-releasing hormone desensitization preferentially inhibits expression of the luteinizing hormone β subunit gene in vivo. *Endocrinology* **122:** 1689–1694.

Levine JE, Norman RL, Gliessman PM, Oyama TT, Bangsberg DR & Spies HG (1985) In vivo gonadotropin-releasing hormone release and serum luteinizing hormone measurements in ovariectomized, estrogen-treated rhesus monkeys. *Endocrinology* **117:** 711–721.

Lincoln GA & Fraser HM (1987) Compensatory response of the LHRH/LH pulse generator following administration of a potent LHRH antagonist in the ram. *Endocrinology* **120:** 2245–2250.

Ling N, Ying S-Y, Uneno N et al (1986) Pituitary FSH is released by a heterodimer of the β-subunits from the two forms of inhibin. *Nature* **321:** 779–782.

MacLeod TL, Eisen A & Sussman GL (1987) Anaphylactic reaction to synthetic luteinizing hormone-releasing hormone. *Fertility and Sterility* **48:** 500–502.

Mais V, Kazer RR, Cetel NS, Rivier J, Vale W & Yen SSC (1986) The dependency of folliculogenesis and corpus luteum function on pulsatile gonadotropin secretion in cycling women using a gonadotropin-releasing hormone antagonist as a probe. *Journal of Clinical Endocrinology and Metabolism* **62:** 1250–1255.

Marshall GR, Akhtar FB, Weinbauer GF & Neischlag E (1986) Gonadotrophin-releasing hormone (GnRH) overcomes GnRH antagonist-induced suppression of LH secretion in primates. *Journal of Endocrinology* **110:** 145–150.

Mason AJ, Pitts SL, Nikolics K et al (1986) The hypogonadal mouse: reproductive functions restored by gene therapy. *Science* **234:** 1372–1378.

Matta WH, Shaw RW, Hesp R & Katz D (1987) Hypogonadism induced by luteinizing hormone releasing hormone agonist analogues: effects on bone density in premenopausal women. *British Medical Journal* **29:** 1523–1524.

McCann SM, Samson WK, Aguila MC et al (1986) The role of brain peptides in the control of anterior pituitary hormone secretion. In Fink G, Harmar AJ, McKerns KW (eds) *Neuroendocrine Molecular Biology*, pp 101–112. New York: Plenum Press.

McLachlan RI, Robertson DM, De Kretser D & Burger HG (1987) Inhibin—a non-steroidal regulator of pituitary follicle stimulating hormone. *Clinical Endocrinology and Metabolism* **1:** 89–112.

Meakin JL, Keogh EJ & Martin CE (1985) Human anti-luteinizing hormone releasing hormone antibodies in patients treated with synthetic luteinizing hormone releasing hormone. *Fertility and Sterility* **43:** 811–813.

Meldrum DR, Tsao Z, Monroe SE, Braunstein GD & Sladek J (1984) Stimulation of LH fragments with reduced bioactivity following GnRH agonist administration in women. *Journal of Clinical Endocrinology and Metabolism* **58:** 755–757.

Millar RP, Wormald PJ & Milton RC deL (1986) Stimulation of gonadotropin release by a non-GnRH peptide sequence of the GnRH precursor. *Science* **232:** 68–70.

Milton SCF, Millar RP & Milton RC deL (1987) LH-releasing activity and receptor binding of pH GnRH 14-26 analogues. *Biochemical and Biophysical Research Communications* **143:** 872–879.

Nikolics K, Mason AJ, Szonyi E, Ramachandran J & Seeburg PH (1985) A prolactin-inhibitory factor within the precursor for human gonadotropin-releasing hormone. *Nature* **316:** 511–517.

Pohl CR, Richardson DW, Hutchison JS, Germak JA & Knobil E (1983) Hypophysiotropic signal frequency and the functioning of the pituitary–ovarian system in the rhesus monkey. *Endocrinology* **112:** 2076–2080.

Ronnekleiv OK, Adelman JP, Weber E, Herbert E & Kelly MJ (1987) Immunohistochemical demonstration of proGnRH and GnRH in the preoptic-basal hypothalamus of the primate. *Neuroendocrinology* **45:** 518–521.

Sandow J (1983) The regulation of LHRH action at the pituitary and gonadal receptor level: a review. *Psychoneuroendocrinology* **8:** 277–297.

Sandow J, Fraser HM & Geisthovel F (1986) Pharmacology and experimental basis of therapy with LHRH agonists in women. In Rolland R, Chadha DR & Willemsen WNP (eds) *Gonadotropin Down-regulation in Gynaecological Practice*, pp 1–27. New York: Alan Liss.

Sandow J, Fraser HM, Seidel H, Kraus B, Jerabeck-Sandow G & Von Rechenberg W (1987) Buserelin: pharmacokinetics, metabolism and mechanisms of action. *British Journal of Clinical Practice* **41(suppl 48):** 6–12.

Seeburg PH & Adelman JP (1984) Characterization of cDNA for precursor of human luteinizing hormone releasing hormone. *Nature* **311:** 666.

Seeburg PH, Mason AJ, Stewart TA & Nikolics K (1987) The mammalian GnRH gene and its pivotal role in reproduction. *Recent Progress in Hormone Research* **43:** 69–98.

Standish LJ, Adams LA, Vician L, Clifton DK & Steiner RA (1987) Neuroanatomical localization of cells containing gonadotropin-releasing hormone messenger ribonucleic acid in the primate brain by in situ hybridization histochemistry. *Molecular Endocrinology* **1:** 371–376.

Vale W, Rivier J, Vaughan J et al (1986) Purification and characterization of an FSH releasing protein from porcine follicular fluid. *Nature* **321:** 766–779.

Vickery BH & Nestor JJ Jr (1987) Luteinizing hormone-releasing hormone analogs: development and mechanism of action. *Seminars in Reproductive Endocrinology* **5:** 353–369.

Waibel S, Bremen T, Schiffl R et al (1988) Bone density in patients treated with GnRH agonists for myomata and endometriosis. *Gynecological Endocrinology* **2(suppl 1)** abstract 96.

Walker KJ, Turkes A, Williams MR, Blamey RW & Nicholson RI (1984) Preliminary endocrinological evaluation of a sustained-release formulation of the LH-releasing hormone agonist D-Ser(But)6Azgly 10 LHRH in premenopausal women with advanced breast cancer. *Journal of Endocrinology* **111:** 349–353.

West CP & Baird DT (1987) Suppression of ovarian activity by Zoladex depot (ICI 118630), a long acting LHRH agonist analogue. *Clinical Endocrinology* **26:** 213–220.

West CP, Lumsden MA, Lawson S, Williamson J & Baird DT (1987) Shrinkage of uterine fibroids during therapy with goserelin (Zoladex): a luteinizing hormone-releasing hormone agonist administered as a monthly subcutaneous depot. *Fertility and Sterility* **48:** 45–51.

Wienbauer GF, Surmann FJ, Akhtar FB et al (1984) Reversible inhibition of testicular function by a gonadotropin hormone-releasing hormone antagonist in monkeys (*Macaca fascicularis*). *Fertility and Sterility* **42:** 906–914.

Wong PC & Asch RH (1987) Induction of follicular development with luteinizing hormone-releasing hormone. *Seminars in Reproductive Endocrinology* **5:** 399–409.

Yen SSC, Lasley PL, Wang CF, Leblanc H & Siler TM (1975) The operating characteristics of the hypothalamic–pituitary system during the menstrual cycle and observations of biological action of somatostatin. *Recent Progress in Hormone Research* **31:** 321–363.

Zeleznik AJ, Kubik CJ (1986) Ovarian responses in macaques to pulsatile infusion of follicle-stimulating hormone (FSH) and luteinizing hormone: increased sensitivity of the maturing follicle to FSH. *Endocrinology* **119:** 2025–2032.

Zorn JR, Barata M, Brami C et al (1988) Ovarian stimulation for in vitro fertilization combining administration of gonadotrophins and blockade of the pituitary with D-Trp-6-LH-RH microcapsules: pilot studies with two protocols. *Human Reproduction* **3:** 235–239.

# 10

# LHRH analogues in the treatment of endometriosis—comparative results with other treatments

## R. W. SHAW

In 1860 Von Rokitanski first described what is now known as endometriosis, although he called it adenomyoma and this term persisted for nearly 60 years. In 1921 Sampson was considered to be the first to define the disease accurately and Blair Bell in 1922 coined the term 'endometriosis' and 'endometrioma'. In spite of these reports, many aspects of the disease, including its pathogenesis, natural history and its relationship with infertility remain obscure. Endometriosis is characterized by the presence of functioning endometrial-like glands and stroma in areas other than the uterine cavity. The diagnosis is best restricted to the finding of such lesions outside the uterus, thus excluding the condition of adenomyosis (endometriosis interna), which is probably an unrelated condition.

The continued growth of endometriotic tissue is dependent upon oestrogen, thus endometriosis is prevalent in the reproductive years with a peak incidence between 30 and 45 years. Endometriosis is the second most common gynaecological diagnosis after uterine fibroids and is encountered in between 10 and 25% of women undergoing laparotomy for gynaecological symptoms in Britain and the USA. The incidence of endometriosis in the general female population is probably between 1 and 2% (Simpson et al, 1980; Strathy et al, 1982) from surveys performed in patients undergoing laparoscopy for sterilization procedures. This compares with the incidence in infertile patients between 6 and 20%. The apparent increase in this disorder in recent decades stems from the more widespread use of laparoscopy in gynaecological practice, particularly in infertile patients in whom this disorder may otherwise be asymptomatic. It is unknown whether the relationship between endometriosis and infertility is coincidental or causal. It is further unknown whether mild endometriosis is an early manifestation of a progressive disease, or whether the natural history is one of spontaneous regression in the majority of patients.

## PATHOGENESIS AND AETIOLOGICAL FACTORS

There have been numerous theories attempting to explain the pathogenesis of endometriosis but no single current theory can explain all the diverse facets of this complex disorder of apparent multifactorial aetiology.

One accepted theory is that viable endometrial tissue may be transplanted by reflux menstruation through the fallopian tubes into the peritoneal cavity or by lymphatic or vascular embolization to distant sites (Sampson, 1927a,b). In addition, endometrial tissue may be implanted by iatrogenic means (usually during surgical procedures) into susceptible recipient tissues, where it may then further develop.

A second major theory is that peritoneal epithelium may undergo transformation to endometrial-like tissue under the influence of oestrogen stimulation with or without other cofactors (Meyer, 1919).

In addition to the above mechanisms, it has been suggested that genetic predisposition and immunological factors may influence the susceptibility of some women to develop endometriosis. Some 7–10% of first- to second-degree relatives of patients with endometriosis have developed the disease, suggesting a family preponderance (Simpson et al, 1980). In addition, specific cellular immunological deficiencies have been reported in some patients with endometriosis, indicating that this disorder may be the result of an autoimmune reaction to an as yet unspecified endometrial antigen (Weed and Arquembourg, 1980).

## SYMPTOMATOLOGY

Symptoms vary depending on the site of the ectopic endometrium. What is apparent is that the extent of the lesions does not necessarily bear any relationship to the intensity of the symptoms and indeed the disease may be an incidental finding during surgery or other investigations for various conditions. Common symptoms related to site are summarized in Table 1.

There has been much controversy over the association between endometriosis and infertility, which occurs in between 30 and 40% of patients suffering with endometriosis (Kistner, 1975b).

**Table 1.** Symptoms of endometriosis related to site of implants.

| Symptoms | Site |
|---|---|
| Dysmenorrhoea, lower abdominal and pelvic pain<br>Dyspareunia<br>Low back pain<br>Menstrual irregularity<br>Rupture/torsion endometrioma<br>Infertility | Female reproductive organs |
| Cyclical haematuria/pain<br>Ureteric obstruction | Urinary system |
| Cyclical tenesmus/rectal bleeding<br>Diarrhoea | Gastrointestinal tract |
| Cyclical haemoptysis | Lungs |
| Cyclical pain and bleeding | Surgical scars, umbilicus |
| Cyclical pain and swelling | Limbs |

The pathogenesis of infertility in patients with endometriosis is poorly understood and is probably multifactorial. With the more severe degrees of endometriosis with obvious anatomical distortions, such as periadnexal adhesions and ovarian tissue destruction by endometriomas, it is easy to explain associated infertility. These mechanical factors can easily interfere with the release or pick-up of oocytes. However, the role of minimum endometriosis causing infertility has been more controversial, with reports of spontaneous cures causing some clinicians to pursue a policy of expectant management in these cases. However, several possible mechanisms have been postulated to explain why infertility occurs in women with mild endometriosis, as summarized in Table 2. At this point in time, no clearcut explanation can be proposed for the occurrence of infertility in women with mild to minimal endometriosis. Some would say it still remains controversial as to whether such cases benefit from any treatment. However, most clinicians would offer therapy to patients if only perhaps to prevent further progress of the disease which may in the future jeopardize fertility.

**Table 2.** Mild endometriosis and infertility—possible mechanisms of causation.

| | |
|---|---|
| Ovarian function | Endocrinopathies<br>Anovulation<br>LUF syndrome<br>Altered prolactin release<br>Luteolysis caused by $PGF_2$<br>Oocyte maturation defects |
| Tubal function | Prostaglandin-induced alteration in tubal and cilial motility |
| Coital function | Dyspareunia causing reduced coital frequency and penetration problems |
| Spermatozoal function | Phagocytosis by macrophages (intrauterine and intratubal)<br>Inactivation by antibodies |
| Implantation | Interference by endometrial antibodies<br>Luteal phase deficiency |
| Early pregnancy loss | Increased early spontaneous abortion<br>PG induced, immune response |

LUF = luteinized unruptured follicle; PG = prostaglandin.

Diagnosis of endometriosis should be suspected in any patient presenting with infertility or with worsening dysmenorrhoea, pelvic pain, dyspareunia or other cyclical associated symptoms related to the bladder or bowel.

For scientific reasons to compare data between various studies it is essential to classify the extent of endometriosis in any given patient. The most widely used classification is that of the American Fertility Society (AFS), first described in 1979 and revised in 1985. This classification, in common with others which have been developed, has some drawbacks in terms of practical application.

## TREATMENT

Endometriosis is a difficult disease to treat as often response to therapy relies on recognition of the disease in its earliest possible stages. In up to 60% of cases following most treatment modalities, recurrence of endometriosis eventually occurs. There is therefore often no permanent cure for the disease and the final resort to surgical oophorectomy in selected cases offers the most effective available treatment. Treatment should be individualized, taking into account the patient's age, wish for fertility, severity of symptoms and extent of the disease. An important aspect of therapy is a sympathetic approach with adequate counselling and explanation to the patient which will also ensure her compliance.

## Surgical treatment

### Conservative surgery

This may be performed in patients with moderate or severe disease when fertility prospects need to be improved or maintained. Procedures performed during laparoscopy or laparotomy may involve dissection of endometriotic lesions, diathermy destruction or laser vaporization, division of adhesions and restoration of pelvic anatomy.

### Radical surgery

When other forms of therapy have failed, and with no desire to preserve fertility potential, hysterectomy and bilateral salpingo-oophorectomy with resection of endometriotic lesions are performed. Subsequent hormone replacement therapy should be kept at a minimum as a small proportion of these patients may develop a recurrence of endometriosis, and combinations of testosterone and oestrogen implants may minimize this risk.

### Medical treatment

Endometriotic tissue has been classically described as being morphologically and histologically similar to the endometrium. In more recent studies using the electron microscope (Schweppe and Wynn, 1981) nuclear oestrogen binding studies (Gould et al, 1983) and cytosolic oestrogen–progestogen receptor studies (Vierikko et al, 1985) indicate that the ectopic endometrium responds differently from normal endometrium to endogenous ovarian hormones. However, ectopic endometrial tissue does respond to endogenous and exogenous ovarian sex steroid hormones in a fashion sufficiently similar to that of normal endometrium to suggest that a hormonal approach altering circulating oestrogen–progesterone levels in the circulation should be beneficial in the treatment of endometriosis. Hypo-oestrogenic states induced by oophorectomy or following the menopause induce atrophy in the endometrium and atrophy and regression of endometriotic deposits. Progesterone and exogenous progestogens oppose the effect of oestrogen on endometrial tissue by inhibiting replenishment of cytosol oestrogen receptors and by induction of 17B hydroxysteroid dehydrogenase which favours conversion of oestradiol to oestrone. Progestogens also induce secretory activity in the endometrial glands and decidual reaction in endometrial stroma in both normal and ectopically sited endometrium.

Medical treatment of endometriosis has undergone a remarkable evolution in the last 40 years. In the past, agents such as methyltestosterone, diethylstilboestrol and high-dose combined oestrogen–progestogen preparations have been used with some success. Therapies which induce decidualization (pseudopregnancy regimens) or suppress ovarian function (pseudomenopause regimens) offer the best chance of clinical remission of endometriosis.

The success of hormonal therapies depends to some extent on the localization of endometrial deposits, with deep ovarian endometriosis responding less well than peritoneal and serosal implants to hormonal therapy.

### Oestrogen–progestogen regimens

Combined oestrogen–progestogen preparations administered interruptedly for 6–9 months were introduced by Kistner in 1959 for the treatment of endometriosis. In more recent years combined oral contraceptive preparations, particularly those with highly progestogenic components, have been utilized, still requiring 2–3 tablets daily to prevent breakthrough bleeding. Side-effects may occur, such as weight gain, headaches, breast enlargement or tenderness, nausea and depression.

### Progestogens

A state of pseudopregnancy can also be effected by the use of progestogenic preparations and a wide variety are available. These progestogens induce a hypo-oestrogenic, hyperprogestogenic state. Because oestrogens are necessary for the process of resorption of necrosed decidual ectopic endometrial tissue, progestogen preparations alone are considered less satisfactory than combined oestrogen–progestogen preparations (Hammond and Haney, 1978). A frequent side-effect of progestogen therapy is breakthrough bleeding together with weight gain, increased appetite, oedema and feeling of bloatedness.

### Pseudomenopause regimens

Danazol is the most widely used treatment for endometriosis. It is a synthetic steroid and an isoxazol derivative of 17 ethyl testosterone. It has mildly androgenic and anabolic properties. The mechanism of action is complex but includes interference with pulsatile gonadotrophin secretion, direct inhibition of ovarian steroidogenesis by inhibiting several enzymatic processes, competitive blockage of androgen, oestrogen and progestogen receptors in the ovaries and endometrium and suppression of sex hormone-binding globulin (SHBG) levels (Barbieri and Ryan, 1981).

The multiple effects of danazol lead to inhibition of the mid-cycle gonadotrophin surge without significantly reducing basal levels of luteinizing hormone (LH) or follicle-stimulating hormone (FSH). A hypo-oestrogenic and hypoprogestogenic environment develops and is accompanied by amenorrhoea and endometrial atrophy—the degree of these effects is dose-related. The use of danazol in the treatment of endometriosis was introduced in 1971; the dose administered being in a range of between 200 and 800 mg daily. Danazol has been shown to be effective in cases of mild and moderate endometriosis (Low et al, 1984) and to induce subjective symptomatic improvement in over 85% of patients with endometriosis (Dmowski and Cohen, 1978).

Post-treatment endoscopic evaluation shows that resolution of endometriotic lesions has been achieved in between 70 and 95% of patients (Dmowski and Cohen, 1975; Barbieri et al, 1982). In a review of pregnancy rates, figures of between 31 and 53% with mild endometriosis, and between 23 and 50% in moderate endometriosis, followed treatment with danazol (Schmidt, 1985).

Danazol treatment is associated with a high incidence of side-effects: weight gain, fluid retention, breakthrough bleeding, acne, hirsutism, oily skin, deepening of voice, muscle cramps, decreasing libido, mood changes, fatigue, hot flushes. The severity and incidence of these side-effects appear to be dose-related but over 80% of women experience some of these side-effects.

Changes in lipoprotein metabolism have also been reported on danazol therapy. These include elevation of low-density lipoprotein and the reduction of high-density lipoprotein cholesterol concentrations (Fraser and Allen, 1979; Cohen, 1980). These changes are reversible on cessation of treatment with danazol at least after 600 mg daily for 6 months.

### Gestrinone

Gestrinone, a synthetic trienic 19 norsteroid, in recent clinical trials has been shown to be effective in endometriosis. Gestrinone exhibits mild androgenic, marked anti-progesterone and anti-oestrogen, as well as moderate anti-gonadotrophic properties. The combined effect of these properties is to induce progressive endometrial atrophy.

The endocrine effects of gestrinone are similar to those of danazol. The mid-cycle gonadotrophin surge is abolished but basal gonadotrophin secretion is not significantly altered. Basal levels of serum oestradiol 17B and progesterone are also reduced. Gestrinone differs from danazol in that it characteristically induces a profound and progressive reduction in SHBG levels by about 85%, and the total serum concentration of testosterone and oestradiol is reduced by 30 and 40% respectively, resulting in an increase in free testosterone index (Kaupilla et al, 1985).

Gestrinone has a long half-life and therefore can be administered orally in doses of 2.5–5 mg twice weekly. Such dose schedules induce endometrial atrophy and amenorrhoea in 85–90% of patients. Controlled studies with gestrinone appear to indicate that it compares favourably with danazol treatment of endometriosis in terms of symptomatic relief and pregnancy rate (Coutinho et al, 1984).

*Side-effects.* In about 50% of patients side-effects include many which are comparable with those seen with danazol such as hirsutism, severe acne, weight gain, voice changes, hot flushes and muscle cramps.

## LHRH ANALOGUES

The possibility of selectively suppressing the ovarian secretion of steroids by repetitive administration of luteinizing hormone-releasing hormone (LHRH) analogues is being investigated as a new therapeutic approach in the treatment of endometriosis in recent years. As already described, surgical castration has so far been the most effective treatment for endometriosis. A reversible means of achieving a medical castration would offer many advantages.

The purification and determination of structure of the molecule of LHRH led to the replacement of amino acids, particularly in positions 6 and 10, producing a series of superactive agonistic analogues which have a reduced susceptibility to degradation by enzymes, and therefore have a prolonged therapeutic action. They have a high binding affinity for the LHRH receptors and continued therapy with these analogues in primates and humans causes pituitary gonadotrophin cells to become insensitive to stimulation by LHRH with suppression of gonadotrophin secretion. This then produces a state of hypogonadotrophin hypogonadism—reversible medical castration (Bergquist et al, 1982). With initial commencement of the LHRH analogues the agonistic action induces an increased output of both gonadotrophins, LH and FSH, for a period of between 4 and 7 days. This increased gonadotrophin secretion stimulates ovarian steroidogenesis but if the analogues are commenced in the early follicular phase this is only oestradiol. When commenced in the mid-luteal phase an increase in both oestradiol and progesterone is induced for a period of 6–10 days. As pituitary desensitization occurs, serum levels of LH and FSH begin to fall; FSH values reach pretreatment basal levels faster than LH. After 7–10 days circulating FSH is below pretreatment values, whereas LH remains at or about pretreatment values. There is an accompanying fall in serum oestradiol 17B (and progesterone when commenced in the luteal phase) with resultant menstruation. These changes are illustrated in Figure 1. The continued administration of LHRH analogues results in low circulating levels of gonadotrophins with no determinant pulsatile pattern of release and suppression of ovarian steroidogenesis. The degree of ovarian suppression depends upon the dose, frequency and route of administration of the LHRH analogue.

The effect of continued administration of LHRH analogues is to produce a medical oophorectomy. The first report of LHRH analogue use in endometriosis was from Meldrum et al (1982) with a small series of five women treated with D-Tryp[6] Pro[9] Net (LHRH) from day 2 of the cycle to assess endocrine response. The drug was administered subcutaneously and the results were compared with a group of 12 women who had undergone surgical oophorectomy and were matched for age, body weight etc. At the

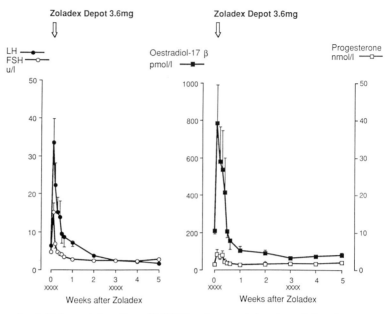

**Figure 1a.** Initial agonistic action of LHRH analogue zoladex depot 3.6 mg in a group of 8 normal women on LH, FSH and oestradiol secretion followed by pituitary desensitization when LHRH analogue was commenced during early follicular phase.

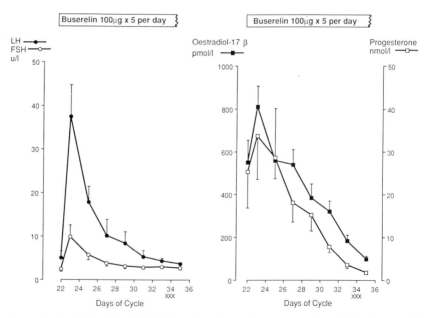

**Figure 1b.** Agonistic action of LHRH analogue buserelin commenced in mid-luteal phase with resultant luteotrophic effect, followed by subsequent pituitary densensitization and luteolysis in a group of 16 normal women.

end of 1 month of treatment serum levels of FSH had decreased below basal levels whilst levels of LH were slightly elevated. In 4 of the 5 patients, oestradiol concentrations had reached castrate range. These hormone levels were maintained to the end of the treatment period. Although the treatment period was short—4 weeks—all patients reported an improvement or even the complete disappearance of their symptoms of endometriosis during that time. Menstruation resumed between 25 and 31 days following the final subcutaneous dose of D-Tryp[6] Pro[9] Net (LHRH). The researchers concluded that a prolonged course of treatment would have similar beneficial effects and this approach needed to be investigated in patients with endometriosis. Since this date many studies have now been published and are reviewed below.

The first definitive report of attempts to treat patients with endometriosis using LHRH analogues came from our own group (Shaw et al, 1983). This study treated 6 patients for a period of 6 months utilizing the LHRH analogue D Ser (tBU)[6] Pro[9] Net LHRH (buserelin). This was administered at a dose of 200 µg three times daily intranasally to 5 subjects and in 1 patient at a dose of 400 µg once daily. The patient receiving the single daily dose of 400 µg continued to complain of endometriotic symptoms, particularly of abdominal pain and her endometrioma increased in size. Treatment was therefore discontinued after some 3 months and the patient underwent surgical treatment. The other 5 patients completed a 6 months' course of therapy and a repeat laparoscopy indicated that the endometriotic lesions had resolved. During treatment ovulation was suppressed in all 6 patients, although detailed studies of urinary levels of oestrogen indicated that in some patients sporadic increase in oestrogen occurred, presumably as a result of some resumption of follicular activity. In some patients these episodes were followed by slight withdrawal bleeding. In other subjects, continued suppression of oestrogen secretion was achieved with amenorrhoea persisting throughout treatment. There were no reported important side-effects with these patients, although some experienced occasional hot flushes. Histological examination of the endometrium performed at the end of the 6 months' treatment phase showed 3 patients with poorly proliferative or atrophic endometrium, whilst the other 3 patients had endometrium consistent with late proliferative development—in these 3 patients there had not been such a marked degree of suppression of oestrogen secretion. In the follow-up period, 1 patient conceived 2 months after ceasing therapy. This paper therefore confirmed the value of the use of LHRH analogues in subjects with endometriosis in relieving symptoms and inducing regression of endometriotic deposits and opened the way for more definitive studies.

A year later a study of 10 women treated for a similar period of time using the same LHRH analogue, D-Ser (tBU)[6] Pro[9] Net LHRH (buserelin) was published (Lemay et al, 1984). The approach by this group of workers was to commence the patients on twice-daily subcutaneous injections of 200 µg for 5 days and then maintain the patients on 400 µg intranasally three times daily for a period of 25–31 weeks. Evaluation of gonadotrophin levels following the initial agonistic increase showed serum FSH had returned to basal levels on the third day of treatment whilst serum LH took some weeks to return to basal levels. By the 30th day of treatment oestradiol 17B levels had decreased below early follicular phase levels and tended generally to decrease over the next few weeks to reach post-menopausal range. An episode of oestrogen withdrawal bleeding occurred in most individuals in the first month of treatment, following which a state of amenorrhoea was induced with only occasional bleeding episodes or spotting being reported in 4 of the 10 women. Symptoms of dyspareunia and abdominal pain were improved or completely relieved within 2 months of commencing treatment and at laparoscopy at the end of treatment resorption of endometriotic lesions to a major degree was observed in all patients. Endometrial biopsy showed atrophic or only weakly proliferative endometrium. On cessation of treatment ovulation returned within a mean of 45 days. Again, 2 of the 4 women conceived between the third and fifth post-treatment cycles. In this study more extensive side-effects were reported, primarily those related to oestrogen deficiency, namely hot flushes and dryness of the vagina. The administered dose of buserelin in the study by Lemay et al (1200 µg intranasally daily) was twice that given in our own initial pilot study (Shaw et al, 1983) and the increased incidence of side-effects probably resulted from the greater degree of suppression of circulating oestradiol 17B.

Our publication in 1985 (Shaw and Matta, 1986) further confirmed the efficacy of buserelin in the treatment of endometriosis. Eight patients were given 200 µg three times daily of D Ser (tBU)[6] Pro[9] Net LHRH intranasally, and 10 patients received 300 µg three times daily intranasally for a period of 6 months. The patients' diagnosis had been confirmed laparoscopically and staged to American Fertility Society's classification prior to commencement of treatment and a repeat laparoscopy was performed at the end of therapy to restage the disease and assess response to treatment. Both dosage regimens reduced significantly the circulating level of oestradiol 17B to mean levels within the post-menopausal range ($p < 0.001$). It was noted that the patients on the lower dose regimen (200 µg three times daily intranasally) showed bursts of follicular activity and rises in oestrogen level but this was seen infrequently on the high-dose regimen of 300 µg t.d.s. With the high-dose regimen (300 µg t.d.s.) some patients reported the side-effects of reduced circulating oestrogen levels—dry vagina, superficial dyspareunia and loss of libido. Hot flushes were also more likely to occur on the high-dose regimen.

In this study, 7 of the 18 patients had some vaginal bleeding occurring between 18 and 38 days after commencement of treatment. In only 4 patients did any further bleeding episodes occur throughout the remaining 6 months of therapy. Symptomatic relief occurred with 11 of the 18 women having mild to moderate dysmenorrhoea prior to treatment, none having symptoms persisting throughout the treatment, and even at the 6-months post-treatment follow-up, in only one patient had symptoms returned as severe as they had been prior to treatment. Five, although having full return of symptoms, were of lesser degree and 5 still had no return of their dysmenorrhoea. Of 6 women complaining of deep dyspareunia at pretreatment, all 6 reported relief of the symptom within 3 months of treatment. In all patients improvement in the AFS scoring was achieved with reduction of

AFS staging. Thirteen of the 18 patients were classified as stage 1 or 2 prior to treatment, and in 12 of these 13 complete resolution of visible deposits was achieved at the end of therapy. The other patients with initial adhesions present remained with significant adhesions since these could not be altered, although partial resolution of endometriotic deposits was achieved and AFS classification improved.

A number of other LHRH analogues have been utilized in the treatment of endometriosis and reports of their effectiveness are appearing in the literature. Schriock et al (1985) reported the effects of naferelin D-(Nal$_2$)$^6$ LHRH in a study of 6 months' therapy with a dose of 400 µg 12-hourly in a group of 8 patients. All patients had prompt and almost complete relief from pain during therapy. A laparoscopy performed before and following treatment in 6 of these 8 women showed complete resolution of active endometriotic deposits. Five patients of the 6 showed only a small single active implant of endometriosis remaining. The seventh patient had a large ovarian endometrioma which decreased slightly in response to therapy but required subsequent surgical treatment. Levels of suppression of serum oestradiol were comparable to those seen in studies with buserelin, reported above, and commencement of the first menstruation post-treatment at a similar time to those with buserelin. On treatment with nafarelin all women developed hot flushes which were extremely severe in 3 patients and necessitated a decrease in the dose to 200 µg twice daily. Following reduction of dosage, oestradiol levels transiently rose in only 1 of these 3 women; the others remained adequately suppressed on the lower dose. Other side-effects were vaginal dryness, transient mild headaches and mild transient depression. In one patient leukopenia developed; no cause was found for this.

Another LHRH analogue IMBZL-DHIS$^6$ PRO$^9$ LHRH was administered to 16 women for the treatment of endometriosis. The dose administered was a daily injection of 100 µg of the analogue; at this dosage oestrogen secretion was reduced to near castration levels during the greater part of treatment (Steingold et al, 1987). Two of these 16 patients treated, however, ceased therapy after 10 and 22 weeks because of emotional side-effects. Thirteen patients had light vaginal bleeding during therapy and all women complained of hot flushes by the end of 2 months' treatment, and indeed 11 patients complained of vaginal dryness. Greater suppression of serum FSH was achieved than LH in therapy but all fell below basal values following the first month of treatment. Calcium excretion was also found to rise to menopausal levels but high-density lipoproteins and cholesterol levels remained unchanged with this therapy.

Our preliminary observations in studies using the depot LHRH analogue, Zoladex*, D-SER (tBU)$^6$ Aza-GLY-LHRH, utilizing a dose of 3.6 mg monthly showed a low incidence of breakthrough bleeding. This compares favourably with D-SER (tBU)$^6$ PRO$^9$ NET LHRH (buserelin) where a significant incidence of breakthrough bleeding has been reported by several workers (Lemay et al, 1984; Jelley, 1986). A state of hypogonadotrophin hypogonadism was achieved with zoladex depot, as well as a more profound and consistent suppression of FSH and LH than that seen with buserelin,

* Zoladex is a trade mark, the property of ICI plc.

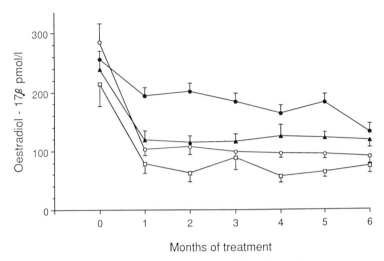

**Figure 2.** Serum oestradiol-17β values in 4 groups each of 20 patients with endometriosis treated with (●) danazol 200 mg t.d.s., (▲) nafarelin 200 μg b.d. intranasally, (○) buserelin 400 μg t.d.s. intranasally, or (□) Zoladex depot 3.6 mg monthly for 6 months.

perhaps reflecting its mode of administration as opposed to intermittent intranasal sprays. Oestradiol levels were consistently below 100 pmol/l throughout the 6 months' treatment period (Figure 2). With the more consistent suppression of oestradiol, hot flushes developed in every patient, varying in both frequency and severity throughout the treatment period and reaching a peak some 12 weeks after commencement of therapy. The more severe hot flushes occurred more frequently.

These studies have been uncontrolled, non-randomized initial assessments of the value of LHRH analogues for the treatment of endometriosis. The findings confirm the drug's efficacy, but comparative studies are necessary to compare LHRH analogues with other established medical treatment. A number of open randomized and double-blind placebo studies have now been initiated and preliminary reports, as detailed below, are beginning to appear from these large multicentre studies. Danazol, currently the most widely used therapy for the treatment of endometriosis, has been the drug chosen for comparison.

Matta and Shaw (1987) looked at the results of a comparative trial in 61 patients entered into a large multicentre study (HRPI buserelin protocol 310 study group). Of the 61, 56 completed treatment and follow-up; 5 were excluded in the treatment phase because of failure to attend follow-up regularly (4), while 1 declined the second staging laparoscopy. Patients recruited were randomized on an open-label basis to buserelin or danazol in a ratio of 2:1. Treatment was administered for 6 months commencing in the early follicular phase immediately following laparoscopic diagnosis, with monthly reviews during treatment, second laparoscopy at the end of 6 months' treatment, and follow-up during the post-treatment period for a further 6 months. Gonadotrophin and ovarian steroid hormones were measured throughout the study together with detailed evaluation of clinical response and side-effects of treatment. Patients allocated to buserelin received 400 µg 8-hourly intranasally. Those receiving danazol were administered with total doses ranging between 400 and 800 mg daily, depending on severity of the disease and subsequent response and tolerance of the drug, according to the manufacturer's recommendations.

Significant hypo-oestrogenism was achieved in both groups but was lower and more consistent in the buserelin group. With the cessation of therapy no residual endometriosis was found in 82% of the patients who received buserelin and in 72% of those who received danazol. These differences were not significant. These figures were based on AFS additive scores of implants alone and did not take into account the presence of adhesions.

There was a significant improvement in the staging of the disease in both buserelin- and danazol-treated patients and a significant and sustained improvement in the symptoms in both groups. Although a large proportion of patients on both treatments developed side-effects, no patient dropped out of the study because of these alone. The common side-effects experienced by patients receiving buserelin or danazol are shown in Table 3. The study indicated that both treatments produced good symptomatic relief, but perhaps buserelin offered better prospects of more marked resolution of the disease when endometriosis was extensive and severe.

**Table 3.** Principal side-effects experienced in patients randomized to receive danazol or buserelin for 6 months in the treatment of endometriosis.

|  | Danazol | Buserelin |
|---|---|---|
| Dose | 600–800 mg daily | 400 µg t.d.s. intranasally |
| Number of patients | 18 | 39 |
| *Symptoms* |  |  |
| Hot flushes | 22% | 74% |
| Breakthrough bleeding | 55% | 23% |
| Headaches | 39% | 20% |
| Vaginal dryness | 5.5% | 23% |
| Superficial dyspareunia | Nil | 5.2% |
| Reduced breast size | 5.5% | 2.6% |
| Weight gain (>3 kg) | 66% | Nil |
| Acne/oily skin | 39% | Nil |
| Mild hirsutism | 18% | Nil |

In 1988 Lemay reported the initial analysis of the total HRPI buserelin protocol 310 study group results and these show comparable results to our own initial subgroup entering that study. Base conclusions were that buserelin has a better efficiency in inhibiting ovarian steroidogenesis and in inducing a consistent and relatively hypo-oestrogen state. At the post-treatment laparoscopic evaluation a greater reduction in the mean score of active implants had been found with buserelin than with danazol, but the relief of symptoms appeared similar with both drugs. The incidence of side-effects was similar in both groups but those reported from the danazol-treated patients tended to be more serious and less acceptable to the patients than those administered with buserelin.

Another comparative study was reported by Jelley (1986); 900 μg of buserelin was given daily and compared with a dose of danazol 600 μg daily in the majority of patients. This study reported excellent compliance and a 7-months treatment period was used. Symptomatic response was comparable in both groups with approximately 60% of patients being relieved of symptoms. Again at second laparoscopy there was a marked decrease in the AFS score in both groups treated. It was noted that the danazol-treated patients commenced menstruation more promptly after cessation of treatment than those on buserelin. No significant alterations in basic blood biochemistry and haematological parameters were noted in the buserelin-treated group, while those patients receiving danazol showed a transient elevation in liver enzymes during therapy. Jelley (1986) reported that some 20% of patients receiving buserelin at a dose of 900 μg daily continued to have irregular menstrual bleeding episodes during treatment, but in these patients endometriotic lesions were favourably reduced despite oestradiol levels not being reduced to post-menopausal levels. Thus the degree of oestrogen suppression required to achieve effective response was questioned.

The optimal dose of LHRH analogue to treat endometriosis was investigated by Minaguchi and co-workers (1986). They studied doses of 300, 600 and 900 μg total daily dose of buserelin and concluded that a dose of 900 μg daily was necessary for clinical effects and suppression of ovarian function, though complete suppression may not be necessary to achieve resolution of endometriotic deposits.

A large multicentre study comparing the effects of $D-NAL_2^6$-LHRH (nafarelin) with danazol is currently underway. Initial reports of this multicentre comparative trial (Henzl et al, 1988) compared the effect of either 400 or 800 μg nafarelin intranasally with danazol 800 mg daily. Placebo nasal sprays or tablets were used in this double-blind study. More than 80% of the patients in each treatment group had improved AFS scores at the post-treatment laparoscopy: mean scores decreased from 21.9 to 12.6 with 800 μg nafarelin, from 20.4 to 11.7 with 400 μg nafarelin, and from 18.4 to 10.5 in the danazol-treated group. All these decreases in AFS scores are statistically significant although there is no statistical significance between the various treatment regimens. Symptomatic relief was excellent on all treatments and similar pregnancy rates have been found in each treatment group after cessation of therapy in those wishing to conceive with an overall rate of approximately 59%. Danazol was again confirmed to induce changes in high-density lipoprotein cholesterol but no changes were observed in the nafarelin-treated group.

LHRH analogues are thus well tolerated effective methods of treatment for endometriosis. Continuing studies are needed to evaluate the long-term effectiveness of these agents with other currently used drugs, both in terms of recurrence rates of the disease and subsequent fertility rates. As LHRH analogues are so effective in inducing a hypo-oestrogenic (pseudomeno-pausal) state, it is not surprising that alterations in calcium metabolism have been reported with increased calcium loss comparable to that seen in the menopause. These effects of LHRH analogues on bone mass (Matta et al, 1987) do present a worrying side-effect; however, the bone loss is reversible at least after a 6-months administration phase. These changes may well determine the duration and frequency of administration of these drugs in the treatment of benign gynaecological disorders, including endometriosis.

It is true to say that as yet there is no totally effective medical treatment for endometriosis but the LHRH analogues offer a further therapeutic option.

## SUMMARY

The induction of a state of hypo-oestrogenism has been found to be effective in the treatment of endometriosis. Continued administration of agonistic analogues of luteinizing hormone-releasing hormone (LHRH) results in the normal menstruating female developing normogonadotrophic-amenorrhoea with reduced circulating levels of oestradiol-17B, often within the menopausal range. Uncontrolled studies reported the efficacy of LHRH analogues in patients with mild, moderate and even severe endometriosis (American Fertility Society classification) following 6 months therapy. A number of large multi-centre randomized open or double blind trials comparing various LHRH analogues against danazol are currently underway. Published results available to date indicate that LHRH analogues and danazol are equally effective at reducing the symptoms of endometriosis and inducing complete or partial resolution of endometriotic deposits. Side-effects are, however, more severe with danazol therapy.

The side-effects experienced with LHRH analogues are those expected from an induced state of hypo-oestrogenism—hot flushes, dry vagina, headaches, superficial dyspareunia—but are well tolerated by patients. The alterations observed in bone and calcium metabolism are comparable to those in the menopause—increased $Ca^{++}$ loss and reversible loss of trabecular bone density have been reported. These effects may limit the duration and/or frequency of LHRH analogue treatment regimens.

The valuable role of LHRH analogues in the treatment of endometriosis has been established and, as newer formulations become available, they are likely to play an increasingly important part in patient management.

## REFERENCES

American Fertility Society (1979) Classification of endometriosis. *Fertility and Sterility* **32:** 633–634.
American Fertility Society (1985) Classification of endometriosis. *Fertility and Sterility* **43:** 351–352.
Barbieri R & Ryan KJ (1981) Danazol: endocrine pharmacology and therapeutic applications. *American Journal of Obstetrics and Gynecology* **141:** 453–463.
Barbieri RL, Evans S & Kistner RW (1982) Danazol in the treatment of endometriosis: analysis of 100 cases with a 4-year follow-up. *Fertility and Sterility* **37:** 737–746.
Bergquist C, Nillius SJ & Wide L (1982) Intranasal LHRH agonist treatment for inhibition of ovulation in women: clinical aspects. *Clinical Endocrinology* **17:** 91–98.

Cohen MR (1980) Laparoscopic diagnosis and pseudomenopause treatment of endometriosis with danazol. *Clinical Obstetrics and Gynecology* **23**: 901–915.

Coutinho EM, Husson JM & Azadian-Boulanger G (1984) Treatment of endometriosis with Gestrinone—five years experience. In Raynaud JD, Ojasoo T & Martin L (eds) *Medical Management of Endometriosis*, pp 249–260. New York: Raven Press.

Dmowski WP & Cohen MR (1975) Treatment of endometriosis with an antigonadotrophin, danazol: a laparoscopic and histologic evaluation. *Obstetrics and Gynaecology* **46**: 147–154.

Dmowski WP & Cohen MR (1978) Antigonadotrophin (danazol) in the treatment of endometriosis: evaluation of post-treatment fertility and three-year follow-up data. *American Journal of Obstetrics and Gynecology* **130**: 41–48.

Fraser I & Allen JK (1979) Danazol and cholesterol metabolism. *Lancet* **i**: 931.

Gould SF, Shannon JM & Cunha GR (1983) Nuclear estrogen binding sites in human endometriosis. *Fertility and Sterility* **39**: 520–524.

Hammond CB & Haney AF (1978) Conservative treatment of endometriosis. *Fertility and Sterility* **30**: 497–509.

Henzl MR, Corson SL, Moghissi K, Buttram VC, Bergquist C & Jacobson C (1988) Administration of nasal nafarelin as compared with oral danazol for endometriosis. *New England Journal of Medicine* **318**: 485–489.

Jelley RJ (1986) Multicentre open comparative study of buserelin and danazol in the treatment of endometriosis. *British Journal of Clinical Practice* **41 (supplement 48)**: 64–68.

Kaupilla A, Isomaa V, Veli I, Ronnbergh L, Vierikko P & Vikko R (1985) Effect of gestrinone in endometriosis tissue and endometrium. *Fertility and Sterility* **44**: 466–470.

Kistner RW (1959) The treatment of endometriosis by inducing pseudopregnancy with ovarian hormones: a report of 58 cases. *Fertility and Sterility* **10**: 539–545.

Kistner RW (1975) Endometriosis and infertility. In Behrman SJ & Kistner RW (eds) *Progress in Infertility*, p 345. Boston: Little Brown.

Lemay A (1988) Comparison of GnRH analogues to conventional therapy in endometriosis. Abstract 020. International Symposium on GnRH analogues. Geneva, 18–21 February 1988.

Lemay A, Maheux R, Faure N, Jean C & Fazekas A (1984) Reversible hypogonadism induced by a luteinizing hormone releasing hormone (LH-RH) agonist (buserelin) as a new therapeutic approach for endometriosis. *Fertility and Sterility* **41**: 863–871.

Low RA, Roberts AD & Lees DAR (1984) A comparative study of various dosages of danazol in the treatment of endometriosis. *British Journal of Obstetrics and Gynaecology* **91**: 167–171.

Matta WH & Shaw RW (1987) A comparative study between buserelin and danazol in the treatment of endometriosis. *British Journal of Clinical Practice* **41 (supplement 48)**: 69–73.

Matta WH, Shaw RW, Hesp R & Katz D (1987) Hypogonadism induced by luteinizing hormone releasing hormone agonist analogues: effects on bone density in premenopausal women. *British Medical Journal* **294**: 1523–1524.

Meldrum DR, Chang RJ, Lu J, Vale W, Rivier J & Judd HL (1982) 'Medical oophorectomy' using a long acting GnRH agonist: a possible new approach to the treatment of endometriosis. *Journal of Clinical Endocrinology and Metabolism* **54**: 1081–1083.

Meyer R (1919) Uber den Staude der Frage der adenomyosites Adenomyoma in allgemeinen und Adenomyometitis Sarcomastosa. *Zentralblatt für Gynäkologie* **36**: 745–759.

Minaguchi H, Vermura TL, Shitasu K (1986) Clinical study on finding optimal dose of a potent LHRH agonist (Buserelin) for the treatment of endometriosis—multicenter trial in Japan. In Rolland R, Chadha DR, Willemsen WNP (eds) *Gonadotrophin Down Regulation in Gynaecological Practice*, pp 211–225. New York: Alan R. Liss.

Sampson JA (1921) Perforating hemorrhagic cysts of ovary. *Archives of Surgery* **3**: 245–323.

Sampson JA (1927a) Peritoneal endometriosis due to menstrual dissemination of endometrial tissue into peritoneal cavity. *American Journal of Obstetrics and Gynecology* **14**: 422.

Sampson JA (1927b) Metastatic or embolic endometriosis due to menstrual dissemination of endometrial tissue into the venous circulation. *American Journal of Pathology* **18**: 571–592.

Schmidt CL (1985) Endometriosis: a reappraisal of pathogenesis and treatment. *Fertility and Sterility* **44**: 157–173.

Schriock E, Monroe SE, Henzl M & Jaffe RB (1985) Treatment of endometriosis with a potent agonist of gonadotrophin releasing hormone (nafarelin). *Fertility and Sterility* **44:** 583–588.

Schweppe KW & Wynn R (1981) Ultrastructural changes in endometriotic implants during the menstrual cycle. *Obstetrics and Gynecology* **58:** 465–473.

Shaw RW & Matta W (1986) Reversible pituitary ovarian suppression induced by an LHRH agonist in the treatment of endometriosis: comparison of two dose regimens. *Clinical Reproduction and Fertility* **4:** 329–336.

Shaw RW, Fraser HM & Boyle H (1983) Intranasal treatment with luteinizing hormone releasing hormone agonist in women with endometriosis. *British Journal of Obstetrics and Gynaecology* **91:** 913–916.

Simpson JL, Elias S, Malinak LR & Buttram VC Jr (1980) Heritable aspects of endometriosis I: genetic studies. *American Journal of Obstetrics and Gynecology* **137:** 327–331.

Steingold KA, Cedars M, Lu JKH, Randle RN, Judd HL & Meldrum DR (1987) Treatment of endometriosis with a long acting gonadotrophin-releasing hormone agonist. *Obstetrics and Gynecology* **69:** 403–411.

Strathy JH, Molgaard CA, Coulam CB & Melton LJ (1982) III: Endometriosis and infertility: a laparoscopic study of endometriosis among fertile and infertile women. *Fertility and Sterility* **38:** 667–672.

Vierikko P, Kauppila A, Ronnberg L & Vikho R (1985) Steroidal regulation of endometriosis tissue: lack of induction of 17B-hydroxysteroid dehydrogenase activity by progesterone, medroxy progesterone acetate, or danazol. *Fertility and Sterility* **43:** 218–224.

Von Rokitansky C (1860) *Ztsch. K. Gesselsch. Aerte* (Wien) **16:** 577.

Weed JC & Arquembourg PC (1980) Endometriosis: can it produce an autoimmune response resulting in infertility? *Clinical Obstetrics and Gynecology* **23:** 885–895.

# 11

## LHRH analogues for ovulation induction, with particular reference to polycystic ovary syndrome

RICHARD FLEMING
JOHN R. T. COUTTS

### INTRODUCTION

#### Polycystic ovary (PCO) syndrome and luteinizing hormone

The capacity of protracted administration of luteinizing hormone releasing hormone (LHRH) analogues (LHRH-A) to suppress the pulsatility and basal concentrations of luteinizing hormone (LH) and follicle-stimulating

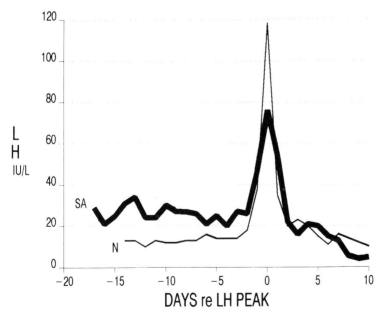

**Figure 1.** LH profiles in a woman (SA) with PCO before and after her LH peak compared with the upper limits of our laboratory normal ranges (N) during the same period. Note that SA shows elevated levels prior to the LH peak and normal levels after the LH peak. A luteal phase sample would have shown normal levels.

hormone (FSH), and thereby gonadal function, has been exploited in therapeutic approaches to a number of problems in reproductive medicine related to steroid hormone production (see accompanying chapters).

Elevated concentrations of circulating plasma LH are common in PCO (Yen, 1980) and this disorder may be unique in that administration of LHRH analogues is targeted directly at an abnormal gonadotrophin profile. The pathological role of LH is complex; not all patients showing ovaries with multiple cysts have elevated values (Adams et al, 1986) and some show variations between normal and supranormal concentrations (Figure 1).

Patients with oligomenorrhoea and PCO show disordered ovarian steroid output related to abnormal follicular steroid metabolism (Baird et al, 1977). This may or may not be caused by the abnormal LH profiles, but the frequent failure of normal ovulation suggests that follicular maturation may be adversely affected by the specific gonadotrophin environment.

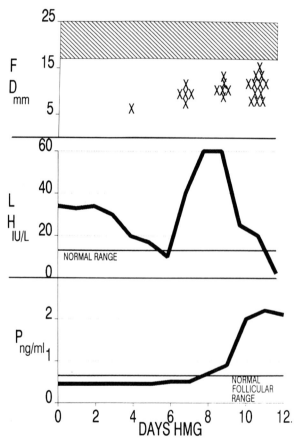

**Figure 2.** Profiles of FD (follicle diameter), LH (luteinizing hormone) and P (progesterone) during induction of multiple follicular growth with hMG in a patient with PCO. Note the occurrence of premature luteinization (PL).

## Problems occurring during induction of follicular growth

During the later stages of follicular maturation in the normal ovulatory cycle, plasma FSH and LH are maintained at low concentrations by the negative feedback effects of oestradiol ($E_2$) and inhibin until the pre-ovulatory surge. By this time the follicle has grown from approximately 10 mm in diameter (FD) to FD = 17–25 mm (Hackeloer et al, 1979) and the plasma $E_2$ concentration has increased to approximately 900 pmol/l (300 pg/ml). This positive feedback surge of LH has dynamic effects upon the follicle by inducing luteinization and ovulation. Accordingly, this event must be precisely timed to coincide with follicle maturity, and the consequences at the ovarian level of a premature LH surge are probably not restricted to an early rise in circulating progesterone or premature luteinization (PL) (Fleming and Coutts, 1986). Evidence for this supposition derives from work in in vitro fertilization programmes where elevated follicular phase LH concentrations have been shown to be associated with poor oocyte and embryo quality (Stanger and Yovich, 1985) and low pregnancy rates (Howles et al, 1986).

Induction of follicular growth stimulated by human menopausal gonado-trophins (hMG) usually results in multiple follicular development. This produces supranormal concentrations of circulating $E_2$ which may have both negative and positive feedback effects. Figure 2 shows an example of this in a patient with PCO in whom the decline and following rise of LH, in the positive feedback surge, was swiftly followed by a rise in progesterone. These effects were observed before any follicle achieved maturity (FD > 17 mm).

This phenomenon was first reported by Gemzell et al (1978) in patients with PCO treated with exogenous gonadotrophins, although it may be expected in any patient with a functional pituitary in whom multiple follicular growth gives rise to elevated $E_2$ concentrations prior to follicle maturity. When luteinization was induced in immature follicles (FD < 17 mm), failure of normal oocyte release was frequently observed (Stanger and Yovich, 1984). In patients with primary amenorrhoea and those with surgically ablated pituitary function, this phenomenon does not exist, and ovulation induction using standard techniques is a highly success-ful procedure (Fleming et al, 1984). The LH surges seen during ovulation induction in patients with intact pituitary function may be suppressed by LHRH-A therapy, reinforcing the case for such treatment of PCO patients.

## LH suppression and consequences

Protracted LHRH-agonist therapy reduces the pituitary secretion of bio-logically active LH and ovarian steroid production in women with PCO (Chang et al, 1983; Fleming et al, 1985a). The LH response profiles differ markedly when assessed by different assay methods. There are considerable qualitative and quantitative changes in subunits (Meldrum et al, 1984) and it remains to be determined if these have differential biological effects. However, immunoassays of 'whole LH' reveal a primary stimulation phase which lasts for 2–5 days, whereupon the circulating concentrations return to pretreatment levels (Figure 3). The subsequent continued decline in concentrations is less rapid and the PCO group, with high levels at the start, require another 10–14 days of therapy to obtain low–normal or subnormal levels.

The initial stimulatory phase can induce ovarian activity (increased $E_2$ secretion), even in patients showing none prior to therapy (Figure 4). This is short-lived and declines in parallel with the LH.

The consequences of LH suppression in patients with PCO appear to depend upon the duration of therapy. The $E_2$ was suppressed to postmenopausal or castrate concentrations by the time LH was fully suppressed (after 12–15 days of therapy), when the androgens, elevated before treatment, were normalized and did not achieve castrate values (Fleming et al, 1985a). More prolonged therapy appeared to be capable of inducing further ovarian androgen suppression to concentrations expected in postmenopausal women (Chang et al, 1983).

## METHODS

### Patients

In our recent study of LHRH analogues in patients with PCO, all PCO patients showed oligomenorrhoea (cycle length > 42 days) with elevated LH

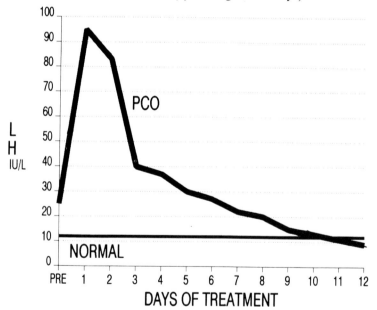

**Figure 3.** Mean LH profiles following initiation of LHRH-A therapy in a group of PCO women compared with the upper limit of normal cycle luteal phase ranges. Although LH levels return to the starting level within 5 days they were not normalized until 11 days.

concentrations and elevated or high–normal androstenedione levels and complained of infertility of at least 3 years' duration. Laparoscopy revealed normal pelvic anatomy and all partners showed semen analyses above the WHO minimum normal standard. Since treatment with clomiphene citrate can be effective therapy in approximately one-third of infertile PCO patients (Macgregor et al, 1968), a minimum of 12 months of anti-oestrogen therapy was required before proceeding to ovulation induction with exogenous gonadotrophins.

## Ovulation induction

Daily injections of hMG were administered until follicular maturity was attained, when human chorionic gonadotrophin (hCG) was administered (day 0). The initial dose of hMG was 2 ampoules/day and daily plasma $E_2$ estimations allowed titration of dose against responses. hCG (5000 iu i.m.) was administered when follicular maturity (FD $> 17$ mm) was diagnosed by

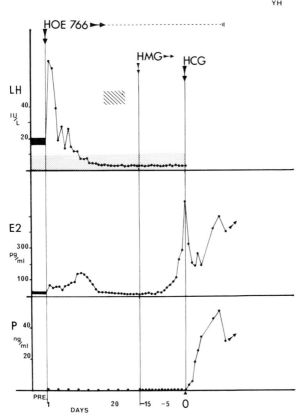

**Figure 4.** An example of the complete course of ovulation induction using combined LHRH-agonist (HOE766)/hMG/hCG therapy in a patient with PCO. This course of treatment resulted in a single conception. The stippled area shows normal cycle LH basal levels and the striped block represents menstruation after the decline of the agonistic effect.

ovarian ultrasound only if the $E_2$ concentration was between 750 pmol/l (250 pg/ml) and 7500 pmol/l (2500 pg/ml). These limits were set to reduce the problems of multiple pregnancy and hyperstimulation syndrome. Further hCG (2500 iu i.m.) was administered for luteal support on days +3 and +6 relative to day 0.

## LHRH-agonist administration

LHRH-agonist can be administered using a number of effective delivery systems, but for the relative short-term and variable duration required for ovulation induction, the nasal spray (buserelin; Hoechst, UK) is both effective and convenient. In this work the most common dose employed was $5 \times 100$ μg/day (Fleming et al, 1985b) although the manufacturers' recommended dose for ovarian suppression is $4 \times 300$ μg/day. Buserelin treatment was started at least 14 days prior to initiation of hMG therapy. As shown in the example in Figure 4, the agonistic ('flare') effect of treatment initiation often causes some ovarian activity, and the ensuing menstrual bleed can be used as a good clinical marker that the gonadotrophins and follicular growth are effectively suppressed.

## RESULTS

### Effects of combined therapy on hormone profiles and PL

During ovulation induction with hMG alone in patients with PCO, a wide variety of LH and steroid hormone concentration profiles can be seen, as the follicles grow towards 'maturity'. PL is a commonly observed consequence of LH rises. In one series of cycles in 45 patients (120 cycles) (Fleming et al, 1987) the concentration of progesterone rose above 1.5 ng/ml (the upper limit of normal on the day of the LH peak during spontaneous menstrual cycles) prior to the identification of a mature-sized follicle in 15 patients (33%). In a similar series of PCO patients on combined therapy ($n = 20$, 47 cycles), PL was eliminated.

Figure 5 shows the LH and progesterone profiles of 13 patients treated with hMG and demonstrating PL prior to hCG administration, and of the same patients treated with combined therapy in a subsequent cycle. The latter cycles showed suppression of both LH and progesterone until after hCG administration, similar to profiles seen in patients with no endogenous pituitary function. The concentrations of $E_2$ were similar in both treatment groups, with mean values of 3750 pmol/l (1250 pg/ml, hMG alone) and 4350 pmol/l (1450 pg/ml, combined therapy) at the time of hCG.

### Conception rates

The conception rates in women with PCO during the first cycle of treatment with hMG alone and with combined therapy in our studies are shown in Table 1. After this the allocation of patients to particular treatment groups

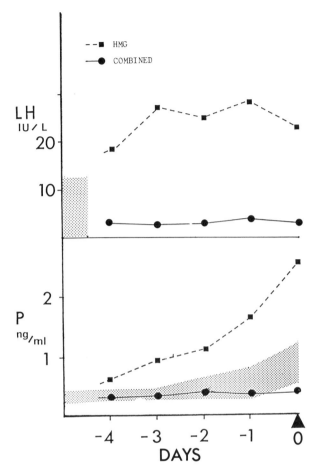

**Figure 5.** Comparison of luteinizing hormone (LH) and progesterone (P) profiles during the 5 days prior to hCG administration in the same 13 patients treated with both hMG/hCG (hMG) and LHRH-agonist/hMG/hCG (combined) for ovulation induction. Hatched areas show LH and P ranges for spontaneous conception cycles.

**Table 1.** Ovulation induction in PCO.

| Therapy | Patients (n) | Pregnancies in first cycle | |
| --- | --- | --- | --- |
| | | (n) | (%) |
| hMG/hCG | 38 | 5 | 13 |
| hMG/hCG/LHRH-A | 40 | 14 | 35 |

hMG = human menopausal gonadotrophins; hCG = human chorionic gonadotrophins; LHRH-A = luteinizing hormone-releasing hormone analogues.

was no longer random. The group on hMG therapy showed conception rates consistent with other published figures, while those on combined therapy showed a significant ($p < 0.05$) improvement to 35% per treatment cycle.

Over a treatment course (maximum of six cycles) this resulted in a pregnancy rate of 78% of patients (Figure 6), approximately double the rates reported for ovulation induction in PCO by other authors (Dor et al, 1980; Diamond and Wentz, 1986; Lunenfeld and Insler, 1978) and in our own experience (14 pregnancies in 99 cycles of 38 patients: 35% of patients). Figure 6 shows that the improved conception rate in PCO patients on combined therapy approaches that which can be expected from women with hypogonadotrophic hypogonadism treated with hMG/hCG.

### Ovarian responses to stimulation

Treating PCO patients with hMG can be difficult because of the problem of excessive multiple follicular development which frequently leads to hyper-stimulation and/or multiple pregnancy (Lunenfeld and Insler, 1978). It was a reasonable presumption that this problem was related directly to the elevated LH concentrations which may increase follicle sensitivity to gonadotrophin stimulation, thus leading to excessive follicular responses (Raj et al, 1977). The reduction of circulating LH by LHRH-agonist may be

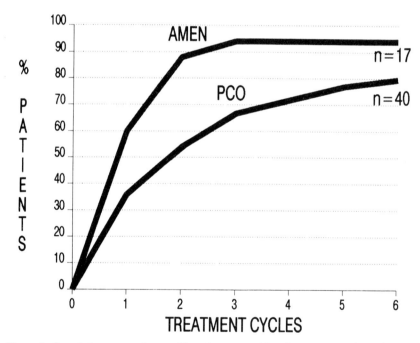

**Figure 6.** Cumulative conception profiles of women with primary amenorrhoea (AMEN) treated with ovulation induction with hMG/hCG and of PCO women treated with ovulation induction using combined LHRH-A/hMG/hCG therapy.

expected to change the nature of this response.

Analyses of the profiles of follicular growth on days $-5$, $-3$ and 0 (within 24 h of hCG administration) in the 13 patients treated with both hMG and combined therapies showed no difference in the rates of growth or the numbers of small, medium, and large follicles observed at any stage. The dynamics of follicular growth were unchanged by LH suppression. The numbers of large ('mature'; FD $>17$ mm) follicles and small (10–13 mm) follicles present on day 0 in the PCO group on combined therapy were compared with those in a control group (normal LH and normal menstrual rhythm) treated identically. There were significantly ($p < 0.05$) more small follicles present in the PCO group. Comparisons of the profiles of follicular development on day 0 in patients with hypogonadotrophic hypogonadism treated with hMG revealed similar data, with the PCO group showing approximately twice the number of small follicles present at the end of the course of hMG (Figure 7).

These data indicate that suppression of LH in PCO patients does not convert their ovarian responses into those expected from patients with hypogonadotrophic hypogonadism, even though the rate of effective ovulation can be improved. This suggests that PCO is a disorder of ovarian function, the consequence of which is high follicular sensitivity irrespective of the circulating concentrations of LH.

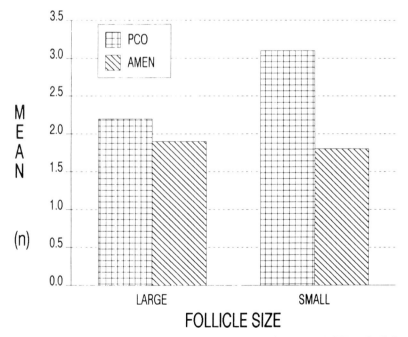

**Figure 7.** Comparison of numbers of large (FD = 17–25 mm) and small (FD = 10–13.5 mm) follicles on day 0 in patients with PCO treated with combined therapy and in patients with primary amenorrhoea (AMEN) treated with hMG alone.

## DISCUSSION

Results have been presented from three groups of our patients treated with ovulation induction: PCO patients treated with hMG alone and with combined therapy; patients with hypogonadotrophic hypogonadism treated with hMG alone, and patients with normal LH and normal menstrual rhythm given combined therapy. All were treated with ovulation induction using the same criteria. The suppression of LH in the PCO group significantly improved the efficacy of ovulation induction and the pregnancy rate. The resultant cumulative pregnancy profile approached that of patients with hypogonadotrophic hypogonadism.

The buserelin therapy eliminated PL and this, the most obvious consequence of LH suppression, may explain the improvement in pregnancy rate. The possible beneficial effects of low concentrations of LH during follicular development may also go some way to explain the improvements (Stanger and Yovich, 1985), but the evidence for this is not yet clearly delineated.

The practical clinical benefits of combined therapy are not restricted to the improved pregnancy rate, since although the incidence of overstimulation ($E_2$ in excess of 2500 pg/ml prior to the establishment of day 0 ultrasound criteria) is unchanged by the combined therapy, the problems of spontaneous ovulation of these multiple follicles is avoided. Under these circumstances hCG can be withheld and ovulation will not occur provided the buserelin therapy is continued.

The evidence from the profiles of follicular development indicates that the high degree of follicular sensitivity in PCO is unaffected by LH suppression. This suggests that the major benefit for ovulation induction in these patients lies not in the correction of the metabolic disorder of PCO, but in the elimination of PL. This results in an improvement of the effective ovulation rate by allowing direct clinical control of the timing of luteinization and ovulation.

## SUMMARY

Infertile women with PCO have been treated with exogenous gonadotrophins (hMG/hCG) for ovulation induction either with or without LHRH-agonist treatment. Those treated without LHRH-agonist-induced LH suppression showed PL in >30% of the cycles and this problem was eliminated by LHRH-agonist therapy. The pregnancy rate (approximately 80% of patients) during the combined therapy was approximately twice that of the group treated with hMG/hCG alone. The suppression of endogenous LH by the LHRH-agonist appeared to have no effect upon the profiles of follicular development in response to hMG, and a high rate of follicle recruitment characterized all PCO treatment cycles irrespective of circulating LH concentrations. These results suggest that LH suppression improves the efficacy of ovulation induction but has no influence on the primary metabolic disturbance in the PCO syndrome.

## REFERENCES

Adams J, Polson JW & Franks S (1986) Prevalence of polycystic ovaries in women with anovulation and idiopathic hirsutism. *British Medical Journal* **293:** 355–359.

Baird DT, Corker CG, Davidson DW et al (1977) Pituitary ovarian relationship in polycystic ovary syndrome. *Journal of Clinical Endocrinology and Metabolism* **45:** 798–809.

Chang JR, Laufer LR, Meldrum DR et al (1983) Steroid secretion in PCOD after suppression by a long acting gonadotropin releasing hormone agonist. *Journal of Clinical Endocrinology and Metabolism* **56:** 897–903.

Diamond MP & Wentz AC (1986) Ovulation induction with human menopausal gonadotropins. *Obstetrics and Gynecology Survey* **41:** 480–490.

Dor J, Itzwic DJ, Mashiach S et al (1980) Cumulative conception rates following gonadotropin therapy. *American Journal of Obstetrics and Gynecology* **136:** 102–105.

Fleming R & Coutts JRT (1986) Induction of multiple follicular growth in normally menstruating women with endogenous gonadotropin suppression. *Fertility and Sterility* **45:** 226–230.

Fleming R, Hamilton MPR & Coutts JRT (1984) Evidence against a high incidence of embryonic loss due to genetic factors. *British Medical Journal* **288:** 1576.

Fleming R, Black WP & Coutts JRT (1985a) Effects of LH suppression in polycystic ovary syndrome. *Clinical Endocrinology* **23:** 683–688.

Fleming R, Haxton MJ, Hamilton MPR et al (1985b) Successful treatment of infertile women with oligomenorrhoea using a combination of a LHRH agonist and exogenous gonadotrophins. *British Journal of Obstetrics and Gynecology* **92:** 369–374.

Fleming R, Yates RWS, Haxton MJ et al (1987) Ovulation induction using the combination of buserelin and exogenous gonadotrophins in women with functional pituitaries. *British Journal of Clinical Practice* **41 (supplement 48):** 34–39.

Gemzell CA, Kemman E & Jones JR (1978) Premature ovulation during administration of human menopausal gonadotropins in non-ovulatory women. *Infertility* **1:** 1–10.

Hackeloer BJ, Fleming R, Robinson HP et al (1979) Correlation of ultrasonic and endocrinological assessment of follicular development. *American Journal of Obstetrics and Gynecology* **135:** 122–128.

Howles CM, MacNamee MC, Edwards RG et al (1986) Effect of high tonic levels of LH on outcome of in vitro fertilisation. *Lancet* **ii:** 521–522.

Lunenfeld B & Insler V (eds) (1978) *Infertility*. Berlin: Gross Verlag.

MacGregor AH, Johnson JE & Bunde CA (1968) Further clinical experience with clomiphene citrate. *Fertility and Sterility* **19:** 616–622.

Meldrum DR, Tsao Z, Monroe SE et al (1984) Stimulation of LH fragments with reduced bioactivity following GnRH agonist administration in women. *Journal of Clinical Endocrinology and Metabolism* **58:** 755–757.

Raj SG, Berger MJ, Grimes EM et al (1977) The use of gonadotropins for the induction of ovulation in women with polycystic ovarian disease. *Fertility and Sterility* **28:** 1280–1284.

Stanger JD & Yovich JL (1984) Failure of human oocyte release at ovulation. *Fertility and Sterility* **41:** 827–832.

Stanger JD & Yovich JL (1985) Reduced in vitro fertilization of human oocytes from patients with raised basal luteinizing hormone levels during the follicular phase. *British Journal of Obstetrics and Gynaecology* **92:** 385–393.

Yen SSC (1980) The polycystic ovary syndrome. *Clinical Endocrinology* **12:** 177–208.

## 12

# LHRH analogues in the management of uterine fibroids, premenstrual syndrome and breast malignancies

## C. P. WEST

The analogues of luteinizing hormone-releasing hormone (LHRH) are a group of therapeutic agents in which the natural peptide sequence of the parent compound has been substituted to give synthetic derivatives with greater potency and longer duration of action. Of the two groups of analogues, agonists include peptide substitutions in one or two positions whereas antagonists incorporate multiple substitutions. When LHRH agonists are given in repeated doses or as slow-release depots, initial and transient stimulation of gonadotrophin release is followed by pituitary LHRH receptor desensitization and consequent gonadal suppression (Sandow, 1983). The antagonists also cause pituitary–gonadal suppression but without the initial phase of stimulation (Kenigsberg and Hodgen, 1986). However, they require to be given in considerably larger doses (Vickery, 1986) and because of the multiple peptide substitutions they are more likely to provoke allergic reactions—a problem very rarely encountered with the agonists. Clinical studies of the agonist analogues are considerably more advanced than those involving antagonists and this review will deal exclusively with the former.

## GENERAL CONSIDERATIONS

### Clinical uses and choice of agonist

LHRH analogues are of potential value in hormone-dependent conditions in both males and females and are now established for the management of advanced prostatic carcinoma (Schally and Comaru-Schally, 1987). They have advantages over other therapies used for precocious puberty (Luder et al, 1984). There are a number of potential indications in women (Table 1). At present, choice of agonist is limited by availability; all have identical modes of action although they have different potencies and methods of administration (Vickery, 1986; Fraser and Baird, 1987). The dose and route selected will vary according to the indication for therapy; this is discussed in greater detail in

**Table 1.** Possible clinical applications of LHRH agonists in women.

Endometriosis
Uterine fibroids
Menorrhagia
Premenstrual syndrome
Contraception
Ovulation induction regimens
Breast cancer
Ovarian cancer

relation to the specific conditions considered in this chapter. The intranasal route has been most frequently used although, even at high doses, ovarian suppression is often incomplete (Hardt and Schmidt-Gollwitzer, 1983). Where greater suppression is required, the subcutaneous route may be used (Klijn et al, 1984; Maheux et al, 1985). The disadvantage to the patient of daily subcutaneous injections has been overcome by sustained-release formulations (Hutchison and Furr, 1987), which incorporate the agonist in a biodegradable copolymer from which it is released at a constant rate for 28 days or longer. Depot preparations currently available are goserelin (Zoladex), administered as a subcutaneous rod from a prepacked syringe (Walker et al, 1986; West and Baird, 1987) and tryptorelin (Decapeptyl) microcapsules given by monthly intramuscular injection (Roger et al, 1986). Such slow-release preparations have the advantage of ensuring compliance and constant plasma concentrations of the agonist.

### Side-effects

While the adverse effects of therapy appear to be confined to those which occur as a consequence of the hypo-oestrogenic state (Fraser and Baird, 1987), they are important in premenopausal women, especially those receiving agonists for benign conditions. Oestrogen withdrawal in premenopausal women is associated with accelerated bone loss (Lindsay et al, 1976) and an increased risk of osteoporosis. Studies of bone density have demonstrated a small but significant loss of trabecular bone in lumbar vertebrae after 6 months' therapy with intranasal buserelin (Matta et al, 1987) although this loss is reversed after cessation of therapy. More information is needed based on larger numbers of women before the risk to the skeleton can be fully assessed. Nevertheless, the problem of bone loss remains the major, if not the sole, contraindication to the long-term use of these agents in premenopausal women.

Vasomotor symptoms are directly related to the degree of oestrogen suppression (Hardt and Schmidt-Gollwitzer, 1983) and are not a problem with low-dose intranasal therapy (Bergquist et al, 1982). However with subcutaneous injections or depots, hot flushes are experienced by the majority of women (Maheux et al, 1985; West et al, 1987) although they have not been a cause of withdrawal from treatment. Vaginal symptoms are less frequent and adverse effects on libido have varied between none

(Maheux et al, 1985) and half (Lemay et al, 1984) of those treated. Other problems occasionally mentioned are headaches, nasal irritation from the spray, irritation and bruising around injection sites and mild skin rashes.

With subcutaneous therapy, amenorrhoea is usual after the initial treatment cycle (Maheux et al, 1985; West and Baird, 1987). For many women this may be a positive benefit of therapy. However irregular bleeding is a problem with intranasal administration (Bergquist et al, 1982; Brenner et al, 1985), particularly during the initial weeks and with lower-dose regimens. It is accompanied by marked fluctuations in circulating oestradiol which raises concerns about the adverse effects of unopposed oestrogen on the endometrium, especially as hyperplastic changes have been reported (Schmidt-Gollwitzer et al, 1981).

### Endocrine considerations

Once therapy with agonists of LHRH is established, ovulation is inhibited (Figure 1c) and gonadotrophins remain at basal concentrations. Ovarian

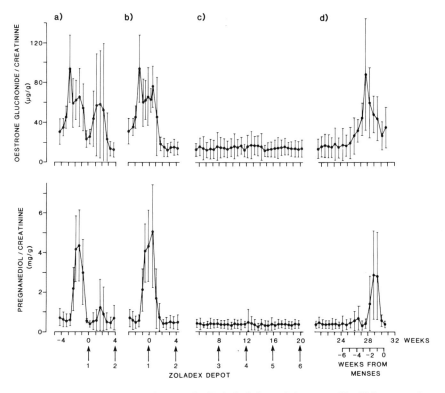

**Figure 1.** Effect of therapy with goserelin (Zoladex) depot 3.6 mg monthly. Urinary ovarian steroid metabolites (mean ± s.d.) measured twice weekly (a) Prior to and during the initial treatment cycle in 6 subjects commencing in the early follicular phase; (b) in 14 subjects starting in the mid-luteal phase; (c) during treatment cycles 2–6 in 17 subjects; (d) post-therapy recovery of ovarian activity (results standardized around day 1 of menses).

oestrogen and androgen production is suppressed while adrenal androgen output is unaffected (Chang et al, 1983). At the initiation of therapy, marked—albeit transient—pituitary–gonadal stimulation occurs. It is thus important to consider its optimum timing in relation to the menstrual cycle. Stimulation of oestrogen secretion is reduced if therapy is commenced in the luteal phase (Figure 1b) compared with the early follicular phase (Figure 1a), although the degree of stimulation is variable following follicular phase administration. Such stimulation may exert adverse effects on the target organ, for example, the disease 'flare' in men with advanced prostatic carcinoma (Schally and Comaru-Schally, 1987). Increased bone pain was reported in two women with metastatic breast cancer (Manni et al, 1986) although the timing of the start of treatment was not stated.

Similar problems have not so far complicated LHRH agonist therapy in women with other conditions. Bleeding in response to the endocrine changes of the initial treatment cycle is more prolonged than normal menstruation although its overall duration does not differ according to the timing of initiation (West et al, 1987). In practice, it is usually more convenient to commence therapy in the early follicular phase of the cycle to rule out the possibility of accidental administration during pregnancy. The initial stimulatory phase is more prolonged with intranasal administration and, where this is undesirable, its duration may be reduced by using the subcutaneous route for the first few days of therapy (Lemay et al, 1984).

Therapy is often referred to as 'medical castration' but this is a misnomer as ovarian suppression is rarely complete with the doses of agonists in current use. With subcutaneous administration of various agonists, some reports gave castrate concentrations of oestradiol (Walker et al, 1986), while the majority found them to be in the post-menopausal (Maheux et al, 1985; Manni et al, 1986) or early follicular phase range (Healy et al, 1986; West and Baird, 1987). Such results are based on assays performed only once or twice monthly and frequent monitoring indicates low-level follicular activity (West and Baird, 1987) in many treated subjects (see Figure 4). Histological examination of ovaries removed surgically following therapy with a slow-release depot (Robertson and Blamey, 1988) showed the presence of follicles at various stages of development although none had undergone luteinization. The long-term effects of LHRH agonists on ovarian function remains to be determined but rapid recovery follows cessation of short-term therapy (Figure 1d).

## UTERINE LEIOMYOMATA

### Symptomatology and conventional management

Leiomyomata (fibroids) are benign tumours of uterine muscle, estimated to affect around a quarter of women, usually during the latter part of reproductive life. Their symptomatology, comprehensively reviewed by Buttram and Reiter (1981), includes menorrhagia, pregnancy loss and subfertility, although they may be a consequence rather than a cause of childlessness.

Fibroids may be asymptomatic, detected only during routine pelvic or abdominal examination, when they have to be differentiated from other causes of a mass arising from the pelvis. Management of symptomatic or large fibroids is traditionally surgical, usually by hysterectomy. Myomectomy is an alternative for women who wish to preserve their child-bearing potential. However it may not be possible to conserve the uterus, depending on the number of the fibroids and their site. The procedure is often complicated by haemorrhage and post-operative adhesions may reduce subsequent fertility (Bonney, 1931; Rubin, 1942).

The reason for a predominantly surgical approach is in part because conventional forms of therapy are ineffective in inducing regression of fibroids. Another indication for surgery has been the difficulty of excluding ovarian neoplasia as the cause of a pelvic mass or as a coexisting lesion where clinical examination of the ovaries is impaired by the presence of the enlarged uterus. The theoretical risk of sarcomatous change has also encouraged a policy of surgical removal. The incidence of this complication is quoted at 0.5% (Hannigan and Gomez, 1979), although others estimate a lower figure of 0.1% (Buttram and Reiter, 1981), predominantly in post-menopausal women.

### Diagnostic techniques in the evaluation of leiomyomata

The widespread availability of real-time ultrasound has to a large extent overcome these diagnostic difficulties. The accuracy of diagnosis of the site, size and nature of pelvic masses has been quoted at between 80 and 90% (Cochrane and Thomas, 1974; Lawson and Albarelli, 1977). Difficulty may arise in the case of pedunculated fibroids, which may be mistaken for ovarian neoplasia (Walsh et al, 1979). Laparoscopy may be helpful in confirming the nature of small tumours and diagnostic curettage should always be considered where there are bleeding abnormalities, to exclude the presence of coexisting endometrial pathology. Magnetic resonance imaging (Hricak et al, 1985) is another technique which is of value in the assessment and measurement of pelvic tumours, although at present it is costly and limited in availability.

Ultrasound measurements of individual fibroids or of total uterine volume can be used for serial monitoring during a period of observation or in order to assess response to medical treatment. Uterine volume measured by ultrasound (Figure 2) was remarkably close to that obtained with direct measurement in a study of 30 women undergoing hysterectomy for fibroids (Lumsden et al, 1987). Many of the subjects had irregular uterine outlines and multiple fibroids.

### Trials of LHRH agonists in leiomyomata

It has always been assumed that fibroids are oestrogen-dependent, a view based on anecdotal reports of enlargement during pregnancy and regression after the menopause. Following the first reported case of successful treatment with an LHRH agonist (Filicori et al, 1983), there have been a

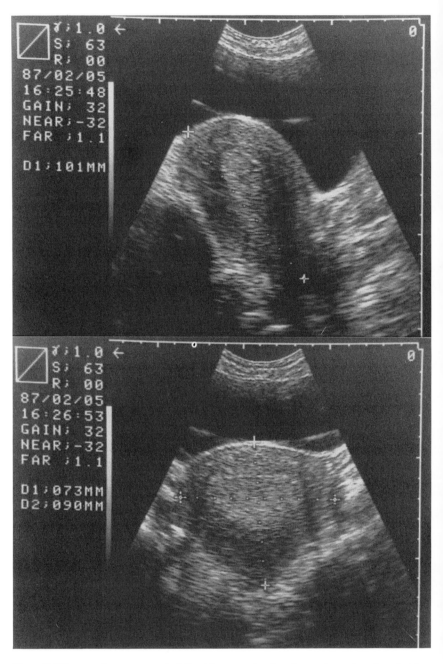

**Figure 2.** Ultrasound measurement of fibroid uterus, showing the maximum length and widest transverse diameters.

**Table 2.** Clinical studies of LHRH agonists in leiomyomata.

| Authors | Subject number | Agonist dose | Route | Measurement | Duration (weeks) | Reduction (%) | Outcome post-therapy |
|---|---|---|---|---|---|---|---|
| Maheux et al (1985) | 10 | buserelin 0.5 mg | daily s.c. | individual fibroids | 24 | variable (0–100) | Regrowth in 6/12 cases |
| Healy et al (1986) | 5 | buserelin 0.2 mg | s.c. infusion | individual fibroids | 20 | 55 | Regrowth to 69% of pretreatment volume |
| Coddington et al (1986) | 6 | histrelin 4 μg/kg | daily s.c. | uterine volume | 24 | 57 | No regrowth |
| Van Leusden (1986) | 6 | Decapeptyl 4 mg | monthly i.m. | uterine volume | 16 | 55 | Not stated |
| West et al (1987) | 13 | goserelin 3.6 mg | monthly s.c. | uterine volume | 24 | 55 | Regrowth to 102% of pretreatment volume |
| Perl et al (1987) | 10 | tryptorelin 0.1 mg | daily s.c. | individual fibroids | 12 | 42.5 | Not stated |
| Friedman et al (1987) | 7 | leuprolide 0.5 mg | daily s.c. | uterine volume | 24 | 53 | Regrowth to 80% of pretreatment volume |
| Friedman et al (1987) | 7 | leuprolide 1.6 mg | intranasal | uterine volume | 24 | 10 | Regrowth to 110% of pretreatment volume |

number of studies of the effects of short-term therapy with agonists of LHRH in women with fibroids (Table 2). These authors have differed in whether they reported the response in terms of the volume of individual fibroids or the total uterine volume but overall results have been very similar. Complete regression of individual fibroids has been unusual with the exception of the smallest tumours (Perl et al, 1987). For individual subjects, volume reduction was significantly correlated with the degree of oestrogen suppression (Friedman et al, 1987; West et al, 1987). Similar fibroid response was seen with daily subcutaneous injections as with monthly slow-release depots (Table 2). However, the incomplete oestrogen suppression resulting from intranasal administration was insufficient to produce a significant reduction in uterine volume. From the practical point of view, administration by monthly slow-release depot is likely to become the method of choice in the future.

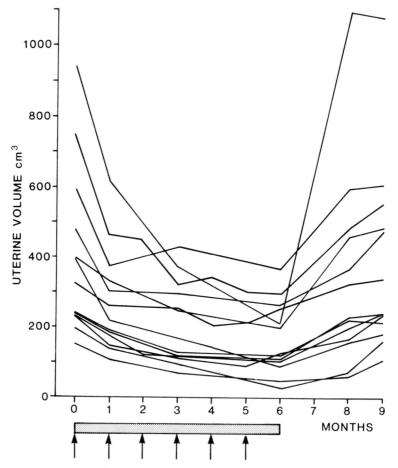

**Figure 3.** Serial ultrasound measurements of uterine volume in 14 subjects before, during and after completion of 6 months' therapy with goserelin (Zoladex) depot 3.6 mg every 28 days.

Volume reduction is maximal during the first treatment cycle (Perl et al, 1987; West et al, 1987) and flattens out after the third month (Figure 3). There have been no reports of the effects of administration of LHRH agonists for longer than 6 months, largely because of concerns about the consequences of prolonged ovarian suppression. However it is evident that shrinkage is reversible and that recovery of ovarian function after cessation of therapy is usually accompanied by a steady increase in uterine volume back to or approaching pretreatment values (Tables 2; Figure 3). This has obvious practical implications, as therapy with LHRH agonists cannot at present offer a permanent cure for the majority of women with fibroids. It will give temporary symptomatic relief and control of bleeding in women who wish to postpone surgery or where surgery is contraindicated, for example in severe obesity. Short-term therapy with LHRH agonists may be useful prior to planned surgery, particularly where the uterus is very large. Significant reduction of operative blood loss has been reported in a pilot study of women treated with goserelin for 3 months prior to hysterectomy, compared with untreated controls (Lumsden et al, 1987). This may also have important implications for women undergoing myomectomy.

**Mode of action of LHRH agonists in leiomyomata**

As discussed above, fibroid regression is directly related to oestrogen suppression and the effect is greatest early in therapy. Significant reduction of uterine blood flow has been demonstrated using Doppler ultrasound (Matta et al, 1987) and this may account for the rapid volume reduction during the initial treatment cycle. It is also important to consider possible actions on hormone receptors in the uterus. Oestrogen and progesterone receptors are present in both normal myometrium and fibroid tissue, with a greater concentration in the fibroids compared with surrounding myometrium (Wilson et al, 1980; Soules and McCarty, 1982; Lumsden et al, 1988a). High-affinity receptors for epidermal growth factor (EGF) have also been demonstrated in fibroid and myometrium (Hofman et al, 1984; Lumsden et al, 1988b) and this together with other related growth factors has been implicated in tumour growth. In a study of women treated with an LHRH agonist prior to surgery, binding to EGF was significantly reduced in fibroids with no change in receptor binding in the surrounding myometrium (Lumsden et al, 1988b). This suggests that the fibroid regression in response to the hypo-oestrogenic state is mediated by reduced concentration of EGF receptors.

Although low-affinity receptors for LHRH have been identified in fibroid tissue, there is no evidence for a direct action of the agonist on fibroids as no overall change in uterine volume was observed in a group of 5 post-menopausal women treated for 6 months with goserelin depot (West et al, unpublished observations). To date, there has been a dearth of studies on the nature of fibroids at tissue level and further research may in time clarify their aetiology and the mode of action of endocrine agents.

## Combined therapy

Despite the benefits to symptomatic women of therapy with LHRH agonists, their long-term use cannot be recommended because of the metabolic disadvantages of prolonged suppression of ovarian oestrogen production. One way of overcoming these problems is to use combined therapy, adding an agent which will protect bone, reduce other side-effects and perhaps act synergistically with the agonist on the target organ. In practice it may be impossible to find an agent which fulfils all of these criteria. Theoretically, the combination of an agonist of LHRH with an anti-oestrogen may act synergistically, as postulated for breast cancer (Klijn et al, 1984), with the anti-oestrogen blocking the effect of residual circulating oestrogen at receptor level. This has not however been confirmed in a pilot study of 6 premenopausal women treated with the anti-oestrogen tamoxifen in conjunction with goserelin (Lumsden et al, unpublished observations). Despite suppression of oestrogen excretion to a level below that reported with the agonist alone, no significant reduction in uterine volume was seen, suggesting that tamoxifen may be exerting weakly oestrogenic effects on fibroid tissue. Symptoms of oestrogen deficiency were however no less severe than in the group treated with the agonist alone.

Another agent tested in conjunction with an agonist of LHRH was the non-oestrogenic progestin, medroxyprogesterone acetate (MPA; Friedman et al, 1988). Again the combined therapy failed to induce significant fibroid regression, despite adequate oestrogen suppression, although the frequency of hot flushes was reduced in women receiving combined therapy compared with those treated with the agonist alone. The dose of MPA selected may have been inappropriate; degenerative changes were observed in leiomyomata during high-dose progestin therapy (Goldzieher et al, 1966). Further studies of combined therapy, including sequential therapy, are required before conclusions can be reached about its value in the management of uterine fibroids.

## PREMENSTRUAL SYNDROME

### Assessment of cyclical symptoms

It has been estimated that severe premenstrual tension affects between 3 and 10% of women of reproductive age (Coppen and Kessel, 1963; Andersch et al, 1986). Most women experience cyclical fluctuations in mood and physical well-being and in up to one-third these are of sufficient intensity to be described as the premenstrual syndrome. The symptoms reported are diverse but most commonly include irritability, tension and depression, with or without somatic symptoms, usually bloating and breast discomfort (Sutherland and Stewart, 1965; Dalton, 1977). A diagnosis of premenstrual syndrome based on retrospective reporting may be misleading (Rubinow et al, 1984). Using daily self-assessment, a difference is found between women whose symptoms are relieved during the post-menstrual week and those whose symptoms persist, albeit at reduced intensity, during other cycle phases. Many of the latter have diagnosable psychiatric problems (Dennerstein et al, 1984). It is important to distinguish between these groups when considering therapy, as only those women whose symptoms are largely confined to the premenstrual phase of the cycle are likely to benefit from hormonal manipulation.

### Preliminary studies of LHRH agonists in premenstrual syndrome

Therapy which inhibits ovulation should be beneficial for women whose symptoms are absent or minimal during the follicular phase of the cycle. A damping down of cyclical symptoms has been reported with the oral contraceptive pill (Herzberg and Coppen, 1970; Silbergeld et al, 1971) although some women with a past history of anxiety and depression react adversely to the pill (Herzberg and Coppen, 1970; Kutner and Brown, 1972). The use of agonists of LHRH in treatment of premenstrual tension has theoretical advantages because ovulation is inhibited without administration of exogenous ovarian steroids and follicular activity is reduced to baseline levels. In a cross-over study of 8 women treated for 6 months by daily subcutaneous self-administration of agonist or placebo (Muse et al, 1984), cyclical symptoms were suppressed after the initial treatment cycle on active therapy. Normal cyclicity of symptoms was preserved during placebo therapy. However the true double-blind nature of such a study is open to question because of the amenorrhoea secondary to active therapy.

The benefits of therapy were less clear in a second uncontrolled study involving intranasal administration of buserelin 0.6 mg daily (Bancroft et al, 1987). Of 20 women who commenced the study, half withdrew within the first 2 months because of adverse effects, usually a worsening of their presenting symptoms. The reason for the high number of adverse reactions is unclear but may be related to the prolonged stimulatory phase seen with intranasal administration of LHRH agonists, particularly when started in the follicular phase of the cycle. The women who continued treatment beyond the second month showed a significant improvement in their symptoms which was related to the degree of ovarian suppression. In some women, irregular anovular bleeding episodes were accompanied by a premenstrual worsening of physical symptoms. Mood changes, when present, were not associated with bleeding.

Administration of an LHRH agonist by monthly slow-release depot has the advantage of more rapid and consistent ovarian suppression. In an uncontrolled study of 11 women with premenstrual syndrome treated for 6 months with goserelin depot, significant reduction of both physical and psychological symptoms was obtained (West, 1988). However, once therapy was stopped, the symptoms recurred at their pretreatment level, in parallel with the recovery of ovarian function (Figure 4). In some individual subjects, low-level peaks of adverse mood persisted during therapy in the absence of ovarian activity, while the physical symptoms of bloating and breast discomfort were more consistently suppressed. These results, together with the observations of Bancroft et al (1987), indicate a dis-

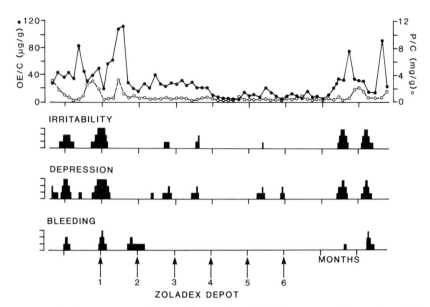

**Figure 4.** Urinary oestrone glucuronide:creatine (OE/C), pregnanediol:creatine (P/C), menstruation and symptom profiles, rated on a four-point scale, in one subject treated with goserelin (Zoladex) depot showing symptom relief during therapy and recurrence in parallel with recovery of ovarian activity post-treatment.

sociation between the physical and psychological manifestations of the premenstrual syndrome and cast doubts on the role of ovulation suppression in its management, even where symptoms are confined to the premenstrual phase of the cycle.

Preliminary results of a second placebo-controlled study (Backstrom, 1986) have supported an overall beneficial effect from treatment with intranasal buserelin. The incidence of adverse reactions was less than in the study of Bancroft et al (1987), occurring in only 3 of 23 subjects. In the study of West (1988), 3 women experienced transient worsening of anxiety or depression early in therapy, following the onset of oestrogen suppression. This suggests that the symptoms were triggered by oestrogen withdrawal.

Results of these preliminary studies of LHRH agonist therapy indicate that pituitary–ovarian suppression may be beneficial in the management of severe premenstrual tension, but in some individuals may aggravate symptoms. Further placebo-controlled studies of LHRH agonists are indicated, both to evaluate their therapeutic role and to clarify the relationship between endogenous ovarian activity and mood.

In practical terms, therapy with agonists of LHRH is undesirable as a long-term solution to a problem which predominantly affects women in their late 30s and which is associated with a high rate of placebo response. However, for the minority of women with disabling symptoms who derive a true benefit from pituitary–ovarian suppression, there is no reason why therapy with an LHRH agonist should not be combined with low 'replacement' doses of oestrogen and progestin, to protect bone and prevent vasomotor symptoms. Such combinations might usefully be explored in future research into the relationship between exogenously administered hormones and mood. As therapy is potentially long-term, the cost would need to be balanced against the severity of the symptoms and response to alternative cheaper forms of therapy such as progestins or oral contraceptives. In severe cases where oophorectomy is considered, prior treatment with an LHRH agonist depot would act as a test of cure before subjecting a woman to an irreversible surgical procedure.

## BREAST CANCER

### Advanced disease—therapeutic options

Breast cancer is the commonest malignancy in women, with an annual death rate of around 40 per 100 000 women (Cancer Registration Statistics Scotland, 1984). Treatment depends on the stage of the disease and the menopausal status of the patient. In advanced disease with distant metastases, the choice lies between chemotherapy and the less toxic endocrine therapy. A randomized study failed to demonstrate any overall increase in survival in women treated from the start with combination chemotherapy, compared with those treated with chemotherapy only after failure of endocrine therapy (Priestman et al, 1978). Ovarian ablation, usually by surgical oophorectomy, is regarded as the first-line endocrine approach in premenopausal women. In postmenopausal women, the anti-oestrogen tamoxifen is the endocrine treatment of choice (Stewart et al, 1980). If there is a relapse after an initial response, further ablative endocrine procedures may be used (Ingle, 1984). These may involve adrenalectomy, hypophysectomy or administration of endocrine agents, such as the aromatase inhibitor aminoglutethimide which inhibits peripheral conversion of androgens to oestrogens (Santen et al, 1974). All these endocrine approaches are associated with a favourable clinical response in around 30% of cases (Ingle, 1984; Henderson and Canellos, 1980a).

### Advanced disease—clinical trials of LHRH agonists

Since the overall response to endocrine therapy in advanced breast cancer is limited, a number of women will be subjected to surgical oophorectomy to no avail. Agonists of LHRH therefore have a potential advantage as an alternative to oophorectomy in the management of premenopausal women and are currently being evaluated in several centres. Recent reports are summarized in Table 3. Of the 132 premenopausal women included in these studies, objective disease regression was observed in 53 (40%), with the disease remaining static in 17%. These results are equivalent to those obtained with oophorectomy.

Once again, the variable and incomplete ovarian suppression seen with administration of even high doses of LHRH agonists by the intranasal route is associated with a suboptimal clinical response (Klijn et al, 1985). The subcutaneous route of administration is therefore preferable in the manage-

**Table 3.** Clinical studies of LHRH agonists in premenopausal metastatic breast cancer.

| Authors | Agonist | Dose | Route | Subject number | Disease response | Disease static |
|---------|---------|------|-------|----------------|------------------|----------------|
| Klijn et al (1985) | buserelin | 1.2 mg/day | i.n. | 22 | 9 | 5 |
| | | 0.8–2.0 mg/day | s.c. | | | |
| Williams et al (1986) | goserelin | 0.1–0.2 mg/day | s.c. | 45 | 14 | 3 |
| | | 3.6 mg/month | s.c. depot | | | |
| Manni et al (1986) | leuprolide | 1–10 mg/day | s.c. | 25 | 11 | 5 |
| Mathe et al (1986) | Decapeptyl | 0.1 mg/day | s.c. | 8 | 3 | – |
| | | 4.0 mg/month | i.m. depot | | | |
| Kaufmann et al (1988) | goserelin | 3.6 mg/month | s.c. depot | 22 | 10 | 8 |
| Wander and Kleeberg (1988) | goserelin | 3.6 mg/month | s.c. depot | 10 | 6 | 2 |

ment of breast cancer. While good results are obtained with daily sub-cutaneous injections, administration by monthly depot is more convenient and ensures compliance. As even these latter methods do not ensure complete ovarian suppression and do not remove the continuing source of oestrogen from the peripheral conversion of adrenal androgens, there is a potential for using LHRH agonists in combination with other endocrine agents. Klijn and co-workers (1985) used intranasal buserelin in conjunction with tamoxifen (5 cases) or high-dose megestrol acetate (4 cases). Numbers were too small to permit meaningful conclusions about tumour response but high and fluctuating oestrogen concentrations were seen in some of the patients treated with the agonist–tamoxifen combination. Those with added progestin showed consistent oestrogen suppression. Tamoxifen when used alone in premenopausal women causes ovarian stimulation (Groom and Griffiths, 1976). The latter problem should be overcome if tamoxifen is given in combination with a slow-release LHRH agonist depot. Preliminary results of its use in combination with goserelin (Zoladex) depot (Robertson and Blamey, 1988) have confirmed the lack of endocrine stimulation, but it remains to be seen whether the combination will achieve improved tumour response.

### Hormone receptors and response to endocrine therapy

A further dimension in the management of both early and advanced breast cancer is the identification of specific receptors for oestradiol and pro-gesterone in a proportion of tumours in both pre- and post-menopausal women. The presence of oestradiol and, to a lesser extent, progesterone receptors is associated with improved long-term prognosis (Hawkins, 1985) and a better response to endocrine therapy (Howell et al, 1984). In the trials of LHRH agonists, both oestrogen receptor-positive and receptor-negative cases have been studied. Response in some of the groups has been confined to receptor-positive tumours or those whose oestrogen receptor status is unknown (Mathe et al, 1986; Williams et al, 1986) while in others, response has been documented in receptor-negative tumours (Santen et al, 1986; Wander and Kleeberg, 1988). These discrepancies may be due in part to methodological difficulties which affect the interpretation of hormone receptor assays (Koenders and Benraad, 1980). Overall, response rates of 55% to surgical ablative procedures in oestrogen receptor-positive advanced tumours have been quoted, compared with 8% for receptor-negative tumours (Henderson and Canellos, 1980b). A similar response to LHRH agonists may thus be anticipated. The response to chemotherapy is around 55%, regardless of hormone receptor status (Henderson and Canellos, 1980b). Thus the use of the less toxic endocrine therapy is justified in oestrogen receptor-positive cases, or where receptor status is unknown.

### Mechanism of action of LHRH agonists in breast cancer

The benefit of LHRH agonists in premenopausal women is presumed to be a consequence of the hypo-oestrogenic state. However, clinical studies of

LHRH agonists in advanced breast cancer have also included small numbers of post-menopausal women (Harvey et al, 1981; Mathe et al, 1986; Plowman et al, 1986; Wander and Kleeberg, 1988). Out of 71 women described in these reports, favourable tumour response was observed in 10%, despite the lack of a significant reduction in plasma concentrations of oestradiol, oestrone, androstenedione or dehydroepiandrosterone sulphate (Plowman et al, 1986). These results in post-menopausal women raise the possibility of direct actions of the LHRH agonists on tumour deposits. Low-affinity binding sites for LHRH have been demonstrated in several breast cancer cell lines (Miller et al, 1985; Eidne et al, 1987). Growth of one of these cell lines (MCF-7) was inhibited in vitro by buserelin (Blankenstein et al, 1985; Miller et al, 1985) and tumour cell growth in vitro has been inhibited by an LHRH antagonist (Eidne et al, 1987). These results support a role for LHRH or LHRH-like peptides in breast tumour cell growth, although their clinical significance is as yet uncertain.

Growth factors are also likely to be of importance in tumour growth and in mediation of the effects of oestrogen. High-affinity receptors for EGF have been demonstrated in breast tumours and in a higher proportion of metastatic deposits than in primary tumours, where their concentration is inversely proportional to that of oestradiol receptors (Sainsbury et al, 1985). Oestrogen appears to stimulate production of growth factors by tumour cells (Dickson et al, 1986). Thus the tumour response to a reduction in circulating oestrogen concentrations may be in part mediated through reduced synthesis of these growth factors.

### LHRH agonists in early breast cancer

Agonist analogues of LHRH are of potential value in the management of premenopausal women with advanced breast cancer. It is also possible that they will be useful in women with early disease. The prognosis for pre-menopausal women with tumour-positive lymph nodes is poor following local therapeutic measures alone, and combination chemotherapy is widely used as adjuvant therapy (Fisher et al, 1975; Bonadonna et al, 1976). Long-term results are superior to those following oophorectomy (Ravdin et al, 1970), but early studies were done without the benefit of the knowledge of oestrogen receptor status. Evaluation of the role of LHRH agonists, alone or in combination with other agents, in receptor-positive tumours is now indicated. A benefit from adjuvant tamoxifen in premenopausal women without axillary node involvement has been demonstrated (Breast Cancer Trials Committee, 1987). However it seems unlikely that LHRH agonists will find a role in this group because of the greater cost and morbidity of treatment when compared with tamoxifen.

### OVARIAN CANCER

Unlike breast cancer, ovarian cancer is not usually responsive to endocrine therapy. However, out of a series of 39 women with advanced ovarian cancer treated with monthly injections of Decapeptyl microcapsules (Parmar et al, 1988), 6 (15%) achieved a partial remission and another 5 remained stable during treatment. Response was not apparently related to tumour histology. Specific binding sites for LHRH have been identified in human ovarian tumours of epithelial origin (Emons, 1988). A multicentre study has been commenced in which monthly injections of Decapeptyl are combined with standard surgical and cytotoxic therapy in women with advanced ovarian tumours. The results of such studies are awaited with interest.

## SUMMARY

Agonist analogues of LHRH are of potential value in the management of oestrogen-dependent conditions in women. However, their clinical effectiveness is a direct consequence of ovarian suppression which is in itself associated with adverse effects, in particular loss of bone mass. They are thus unsuitable for long-term use in premenopausal women with benign conditions but in future may have a wider role in combination with other agents.

In women with uterine fibroids, therapy leads to reduction of uterine volume and alleviation of symptoms although the benefit is rapidly reversed when therapy ceases. Although there is a theoretical potential for combined therapy, successful combinations have yet to be identified. Thus, at the present time, agonists of LHRH do not offer a true alternative to surgery for the majority of women. They will be of value where there is a contra-indication to surgery and for women approaching the age of the natural menopause. They may also be of use prior to surgery, both in controlling symptoms and in reducing surgical morbidity and blood loss.

LHRH agonists appear to be beneficial in the management of some women with severe premenstrual tension but intensify symptoms in others. Particular care is required in selection of women for such therapy because of the uncertain nature of the condition and its high rate of response to placebo therapy. Response is dependent on the degree of ovarian suppression and long-term use of LHRH agonists alone is clearly undesirable. However LHRH agonists alone or in combination with ovarian steroids are of potential value as a research tool.

In premenopausal women with advanced breast cancer, concerns about the long-term effects of therapy with LHRH agonists are less important and these drugs offer a medical alternative to oophorectomy as first-line treatment in women with oestrogen receptor-positive tumours. Future developments are likely to include evaluation of combined therapy and comparative studies in women with early disease. As such studies involve long-term treatment, they will generate very useful information about the effects of therapy. This will be of great value to clinicians evaluating the role of LHRH agonists in the management of benign conditions.

## REFERENCES

Andersch C, Wendestam L, Hahn L & Ohman R (1986) Premenstrual complaints. 1. Prevalence of premenstrual symptoms in a Swedish urban population. *Journal of Psychosomatic Obstetrics and Gynecology* 5: 39–49.

Backstrom T (1986) Buserelin and premenstrual syndrome. *British Journal of Clinical Practice* 41 (supplement 48): 49–52.

Bancroft J, Boyle H, Warner P & Fraser HM (1987) The use of an LHRH agonist, buserelin, in the long term management of premenstrual syndromes. *Clinical Endocrinology* 27: 171–182.

Bergquist C, Nillius SJ & Wide L (1982) Intranasal LHRH agonist treatment for inhibition of ovulation in women: clinical aspects. *Clinical Endocrinology* 17: 91–98.

Blankenstein MA, Henkelman MS & Klijn JG (1985) Direct inhibitory effect of a luteinizing-hormone releasing hormone agonist on MCF-7 human breast cancer cells. *European Journal of Cancer and Clinical Oncology* 21: 1493–1499.

Bonadonna G, Brusamolino E, Valagussa P et al (1976) Combination chemotherapy as an adjuvant treatment in operable breast cancer. *New England Journal of Medicine* 294: 405–410.

Bonney V (1931) The technique and results of myomectomy. *Lancet* i: 171–177.

Breast Cancer Trials Committee, Scottish Cancer Trials Office (MRC) (1987) Adjuvant tamoxifen in the management of operable breast cancer: the Scottish trial. *Lancet* ii: 171–175.

Brenner PF, Shoupe D & Mishell DR (1985) Ovulation inhibition with nafarelin acetate nasal administration for 6 months. *Contraception* 32: 531–551.

Buttram VC & Reiter RC (1981) Uterine leiomyomata: etiology, symptomatology and management. *Fertility and Sterility* 36: 433–445.

Chang RJ, Laufer LR, Meldrum DR et al (1983) Steroid secretion in polycystic ovarian disease after ovarian suppression by a long-acting gonadotropin-releasing hormone agonist. *Journal of Clinical Endocrinology and Metabolism* 56: 897–903.

Cochrane WJ & Thomas MA (1974) Ultrasound diagnosis of gynecologic pelvic masses. *Radiology* 110: 649–654.

Coddington CC, Collins RL, Shawker TH et al (1986) Long-acting gonadotrophin hormone-releasing hormone analog used to treat uteri. *Fertility and Sterility* 45: 624–629.

Coppen A & Kessel N (1963) Menstruation and personality. *British Journal of Psychiatry* 109: 711–721.

Dalton K (1977) *The Premenstrual Syndrome and Progesterone Therapy*. London: William Heineman Medical Books.

Dennerstein L, Spencer-Gardner C, Brown JB, Smith MA & Burrows GD (1984) Premenstrual tension—hormone profiles. *Journal of Psychosomatic Obstetrics and Gynecology* 3: 37–51.

Dickson RB, Huff KK, Spencer EM & Lippman ME (1986) Induction of epidermal growth factor-related polypeptides by 17B-oestradiol in MCF-7 human breast cancer cells. *Endocrinology* 118: 138–141.

Eidne KA, Flanagan CA, Harris NS & Millar RP (1987) Gonadotropin-releasing hormone (GnRH)-binding sites in human breast cancer cell lines and inhibitory effects of GnRH antagonists. *Journal of Clinical Endocrinology and Metabolism* 64: 425–432.

Emons G (1988) The use of GnRH analogues in ovarian cancer. *Gynecological Endocrinology* 2 (supplement 1): 38.

Filicori M, Hall DA, Loughlin JS et al (1983) A conservative approach to the management of uterine leiomyomata: pituitary desensitisation by a luteinizing hormone-releasing hormone analogue. *American Journal of Obstetrics and Gynecology* 147: 726–727.

Fisher B, Carbone P, Economou S et al (1975) L-phenylalanine mustard (L-Pam) in the management of primary breast cancer. A report of early findings. *New England Journal of Medicine* 292: 117–122.

Fraser HM & Baird DT (1987) Clinical applications of LHRH analogues. *Clinical Endocrinology and Metabolism* 1: 43–70.

Friedman AJ, Barbieri RL, Benacerraf BR & Schiff I (1987) Treatment of leiomyomata with intranasal or subcutaneous leuprolide, a gonadotropin-releasing hormone agonist. *Fertility and Sterility* 48: 560–564.

Friedman AJ, Barbieri RL, Doubilet PM, Fine C & Schiff I (1988) A randomised double-blind trial of a gonadotropin releasing-hormone agonist (leuprolide) with or without medroxy-progesterone acetate in the treatment of leiomyomata uteri. *Gynecological Endocrinology* **2 (supplement 1):** 90.

Goldzieher JW, Maqueo M, Ricard L, Aguilar JA & Canales E (1966) Induction of degenerative changes in uterine myomas by high dose progestin therapy. *American Journal of Obstetrics and Gynecology* **96:** 1078–1087.

Groom GV & Griffiths K (1976) Effect of the antioestrogen tamoxifen on plasma levels of luteinizing hormone, follicle stimulating hormone, prolactin, oestradiol and progesterone in normal pre-menopausal women. *Journal of Endocrinology* **70:** 421–428.

Hannigan EV & Gomez LG (1979) Uterine leiomyosarcoma: a review of prognostic clinical and pathological features. *American Journal of Obstetrics and Gynecology* **134:** 557.

Hardt W & Schmidt-Gollwitzer M (1983) Sustained gonadal suppression in fertile women with the LHRH agonist buserelin. *Clinical Endocrinology* **19:** 613–617.

Harvey HA, Lipton A, Santen RJ et al (1981) Phase II study of a gonadotropin-releasing hormone analogue (Leuprolide) in postmenopausal advanced breast cancer. *Proceedings of the American Association of Cancer Research and the American Society of Clinical Oncology* **22:** 444.

Hawkins RA (1985) Receptors in the management of breast cancer. *British Journal of Hospital Medicine* **34:** 160–164.

Healy DL, Lawson SR, Abbott M, Baird DT & Fraser HM (1986) Towards removing uterine fibroids without surgery: subcutaneous infusion of a luteinizing hormone-releasing hormone agonist commencing in the luteal phase. *Journal of Clinical Endocrinology and Metabolism* **63:** 619–625.

Henderson IC & Canellos P (1980a) Cancer of the breast. The past decade. *New England Journal of Medicine* **302:** 17–30.

Henderson IC & Canellos P (1980b) Cancer of the breast. The past decade. *New England Journal of Medicine* **302:** 78–90.

Herzberg B & Coppen A (1970) Changes in psychological symptoms in women taking oral contraceptives. *British Journal of Psychiatry* **116:** 161–164.

Hofman GE, Rao CHV, Barrows GH, Schutz GS & Sanfilippo JS (1984) Binding sites for epidermal growth factor in human uterine tissue and leiomyomas. *Journal of Clinical Endocrinology and Metabolism* **58:** 880–884.

Howell A, Barnes DM, Hartland RNL et al (1984) Steroid-hormone receptors and survival after first relapse in breast cancer. *Lancet* **i:** 588–591.

Hricak H, Lacey C, Schriock E et al (1985) Gynecologic masses: value of magnetic resonance imaging. *American Journal of Obstetrics and Gynecology* **153:** 31–37.

Hutchison FG & Furr BJA (1987) Sustained release formulations of LHRH analogues. In Furr BJA & Wakeling AE (eds) *Pharmacology and Clinical Uses of Inhibitors of Hormone Secretion and Action*, pp 409–431. London: Baillière Tindall.

Ingle JN (1984) Additive hormonal therapy in women with advanced breast cancer. *Cancer* **53:** 766–777.

Kaufmann M, Schmid L & Schachner-Wunschmann E (1988) Zoladex as GnRH-agonist in premenopausal patients with metastatic breast cancer. *Gynecological Endocrinology* **2 (supplement 1):** 133.

Kenigsberg D & Hodgen GD (1986) Ovulation inhibition by administration of weekly gonadotropin-releasing hormone antagonist. *Journal of Clinical Endocrinology and Metabolism* **62:** 734–738.

Klijn JGM, deJong FH, Blankenstein MA et al (1984) Anti-tumor and endocrine effects of chronic LHRH agonist treatment (buserelin) with or without tamoxifen in premenopausal metastatic breast cancer. *Breast Cancer Research and Treatment* **4:** 209–220.

Klijn JMG, deJong FH, Lamberts SWJ & Blankenstein MA (1985) LHRH-agonist treatment in clinical and experimental human breast cancer. *Journal of Steroid Biochemistry* **23:** 867–873.

Koenders T & Benraad TJ (1980) Quality control of estrogen receptor assays in the Netherlands. *Breast Cancer Research and Treatment* **3:** 255–266.

Kutner SJ & Brown WL (1972) History of depression as a risk factor for depression with oral contraceptives and discontinuance. *Journal of Nervous and Mental Diseases* **155:** 163–169.

Lawson TL & Albarelli JN (1977) Diagnosis of gynecologic pelvic masses by gray scale ultrasonography: analysis of specificity and accuracy. *American Journal of Roentgenology* **128:** 1003–1006.

Lemay A, Maheux R, Faure N, Clement J & Fazekas ATA (1984) Reversible hypogonadism induced by a luteinizing hormone-releasing hormone (LH-RH) agonist (buserelin) as a new therapeutic approach for endometriosis. *Fertility and Sterility* **41:** 863–871.

Lindsay R, Hart DM, Aitken JM, MacDonald EB, Anderson JB & Clarke AC (1976) Long term prevention of postmenopausal osteoporosis by oestrogen. *Lancet* **i:** 1038–1041.

Luder AS, Holland FJ, Costigan DC et al (1984) Intranasal and subcutaneous treatment of central precocious puberty in both sexes with a long acting analog of luteinizing hormone releasing hormone. *Journal of Endocrinology and Metabolism* **58:** 966–972.

Lumsden MA, West CP & Baird DT (1987) Goserelin therapy before surgery for uterine fibroids. *Lancet* **i:** 36–37.

Lumsden MA, West CP, Rumgay L, Bramley TA & Baird DT (1988a) Change in receptors for oestradiol, progesterone and EGF in uterine fibromyomata following treatment with goserelin (Zoladex ICI). *Gynecological Endocrinology* **2 (supplement 1):** 27.

Lumsden MA, West CP, Bramley T, Rumgay L & Baird DT (1988b) The binding of EGF to the human uterus and leiomyomata in women rendered hypo-oestrogenic by continuous administration of a LHRH agonist. *British Journal of Obstetrics and Gynaecology* (in press).

Maheux R, Guilloteau C, Lemay A, Bastide A & Fazekas ATA (1985) Luteinizing hormone-releasing hormone agonist and uterine leiomyoma: a pilot study. *American Journal of Obstetrics and Gynecology* **152:** 1034–1039.

Manni A, Santen R, Harvey H, Lipton A & Max D (1986) Treatment of breast cancer with gonadotropin-releasing hormone. *Endocrine Reviews* **7:** 89–94.

Mathe G, Keiling R, VoVan ML et al (1986) Phase II trial of D-Trp[6]-LH-RH in advanced breast cancer. *European Journal of Cancer and Clinical Oncology* **22:** 723.

Matta WH, Shaw RW, Hesp R & Katz D (1987) Hypogonadism induced by luteinizing hormone releasing hormone analogues: effects on bone density in premenopausal women. *British Medical Journal* **294:** 1523–1524.

Miller WR, Scott WN, Morris R, Fraser HM & Sharpe RM (1985) Growth of human breast cancer cells inhibited by a luteinizing hormone-releasing hormone agonist. *Nature* **313:** 231–233.

Muse KN, Cetel NS, Flutterman LA & Yen SSC (1984) The premenstrual syndrome: effects of 'medical oophorectomy'. *New England Journal of Medicine* **311:** 1345–1349.

Parmar H, Rustin G, Lightman SL et al (1988) Response to D-Trp-6-luteinising hormone releasing hormone (Decapeptyl) microcapsules in advanced ovarian cancer. *British Medical Journal* **296:** 1229.

Perl V, Marquez J, Schally AV et al (1987) Treatment of leiomyomata uteri with D-Trp[6]-luteinizing hormone-releasing hormone. *Fertility and Sterility* **48:** 383–389.

Plowman PN, Nicholson RI & Walker KJ (1986) Remission of postmenopausal breast cancer during treatment with the luteinising hormone releasing hormone agonist ICI 118630. *British Journal of Cancer* **54:** 903–909.

Priestman T, Baum M, Jones V & Forbes J (1978) Treatment and survival in advanced breast cancer. *British Medical Journal* **ii:** 1673–1674.

Ravdin RG, Lewison EF, Slack NH, Gardner B, State D & Fisher B (1970) Results of a clinical trial concerning the worth of prophylactic oophorectomy for breast cancer. *Surgery, Gynecology and Obstetrics* **131:** 1055–1064.

Robertson JFR & Blamey RW (1988) GnRH analogues in breast cancer. *Gynecological Endocrinology* **2 (supplement 1):** 50.

Roger M, Chaussain JL, Berlier P et al (1986) Long term treatment of male and female precocious puberty by periodic administration of a long-acting preparation of D-Trp[6]-luteinizing hormone-releasing hormone microcapsules. *Journal of Clinical Endocrinology and Metabolism* **62:** 670–677.

Rubin IC (1942) Progress in myomectomy: surgical measures and diagnostic aids favoring lower morbidity and mortality. *American Journal of Obstetrics and Gynecology* **44:** 196–212.

Rubinow DR, Roy Byrne P, Hoban MC, Gold PW & Post RM (1984) Prospective assessment of menstrually related mood disorders. *American Journal of Psychiatry* **141:** 684–686.

Sainsbury JRC, Farndon JR, Sherbet GV & Harris AL (1985) Epidermal-growth-factor receptors and oestrogen receptors in human breast cancer. *Lancet* i: 364–366.

Sandow J (1983) Clinical applications of LHRH and its analogues. *Clinical Endocrinology* 18: 571–592.

Santen RJ, Lipton A & Kendall J (1974) Successful medical adrenalectomy with amino-glutethimide: role of altered drug metabolism. *Journal of the American Medical Association* 230: 1661–1665.

Santen RJ, Manni A & Harvey H (1986) Gonadotropin releasing hormone (GnRH) analogs in the treatment of breast and prostatic carcinoma. *Breast Cancer Research and Treatment* 7: 129–145.

Schally AV & Comaru-Schally AM (1987) Use of luteinizing hormone releasing hormone analogs in the treatment of hormone-dependent tumors. *Seminars in Reproductive Endocrinology* 5: 389–398.

Schmidt-Gollwitzer M, Hardt W, Schmidt-Gollwitzer K, von der Ohe M & Nevinny-Stickel J (1981) Influence of the LH-RH analogue buserelin on cyclic ovarian function and on endometrium. A new approach to fertility control? *Contraception* 23: 187–195.

Scottish Cancer Registration Scheme (1984) *Cancer Registration Statistics, Scotland 1971–80*. Scottish Health Service Common Services Agency, Information Services Division. Glasgow: McKay and Inglis.

Silbergeld S, Brast N & Noble EP (1971) The menstrual cycle: a double blind study of symptoms, moods and behaviour and biochemical variables using enovid and placebo. *Psychosomatic Medicine* 33: 411–428.

Soules MR & McCarty KS (1982) Leiomyomas: steroid receptor content. Variation within normal menstrual cycles. *American Journal of Obstetrics and Gynecology* 143: 6–11.

Stewart HJ, Forrest APM, Gunn JM et al (1980) The tamoxifen trial—a double blind comparison with stilboestrol in post-menopausal women with advanced breast cancer. *European Journal of Cancer and Clinical Oncology* (**supplement 1**): 83–88.

Sutherland H & Stewart I (1965) A critical analysis of the premenstrual tension syndrome. *Lancet* i: 1180–1183.

Van Leusden H (1986) Rapid reduction of uterine myomas after short-term treatment with microencapsulated D-Trp6-LHRH. *Lancet* ii: 1213.

Vickery BH (1986) Comparison of the potential for therapeutic utilities with gonadotropin-releasing hormone agonists and antagonists. *Endocrine Reviews* 7: 115–124.

Walker KJ, Turkes A, Williams MR, Blamey RW & Nicholson RI (1986) Preliminary endocrinological evaluation of a sustained release formulation of the LH-releasing hormone agonist D-ser(But)[6] Azgly[10] LHRH in premenopausal women with advanced breast cancer. *Journal of Endocrinology* 111: 349–353.

Walsh JW, Taylor KJW, Wasson JFMcL, Schwartz PE & Rosenfield AT (1979) Gray-scale ultrasound in 204 proven gynaecological masses: accuracy and specific diagnostic criteria. *Radiology* 130: 391–397.

Wander H-E & Kleeberg UR (1988) Zoladex—a synthetic GnRH analogue in the treatment of pre and postmenopausal advanced breast cancer. *Gynecological Endocrinology* 2 (**supplement 1**): 137.

West CP (1988) Zoladex depot (goserelin) in the assessment and management of premenstrual problems—a pilot study. *Gynecological Endocrinology* 2 (**supplement 1**): 182.

West CP & Baird DT (1987) Suppression of ovarian activity by Zoladex depot (ICI 118630), a long-acting luteinizing hormone releasing hormone agonist analogue. *Clinical Endocrinology* 26: 213–220.

West CP, Lumsden MA, Lawson S, Williamson J & Baird DT (1987) Shrinkage of uterine fibroids during therapy with goserelin (Zoladex): a luteinizing hormone-releasing hormone agonist administered as a monthly subcutaneous depot. *Fertility and Sterility* 48: 45–51.

Williams MR, Walker KJ, Turkes A, Blamey RW & Nicholson RI (1986) The use of an LHRH agonist (ICI 118630, Zoladex) in advanced premenopausal breast cancer. *British Journal of Cancer* 53: 629–636.

Wilson EA, Yang F & Rees ED (1980) Estradiol and progesterone binding in uterine leiomyomata and in normal uterine tissues. *Obstetrics and Gynecology* 55: 20–24.

# 13

Future directions: anti-hormones in
reproductive medicine

KENNETH A. STEINGOLD
GARY D. HODGEN

Anti-hormones for use in gynaecology and reproductive medicine currently
have a key role, both in clinical management and in the basic research of
reproductive endocrinology. Previous contributions in this book have
addressed specific issues related to particular anti-hormones. Here, our
purpose is to address an overview projecting the anticipated directions of
anti-hormone research and their nascent clinical applications.

## ANTI-OESTROGENS

Anti-oestrogens are useful both in reproduction management and in the
treatment of gynaecological malignancies. In this section we address anti-
oestrogens as they relate to ovulation induction and infertility, their use as
an anti-cancer modality, and potential replacement therapy during menopause.

For most practitioners, the anti-oestrogen clomiphene citrate (CC) is the
predominant drug used for ovulation induction. CC has a reported ovulation
rate of approximately 80%; however, most studies state that only a 40–50%
pregnancy rate is achieved during three or four courses of treatment, despite
apparently normal ovulation (Rabau et al, 1967; Lobo et al, 1982). This
discrepancy has long been a source of concern for clinicians and has limited
the utility of this otherwise efficacious drug.

One proposed aetiology for decreased fertility in these patients is the
increased incidence of luteal phase deficiency (Garcia et al, 1977). This
deficiency may be a result of either aberrant folliculogenesis or an endometrial defect. Older studies reported the decreased steroidogenic capa-
bility of human corpus luteum slices exposed to CC (Sammerstein, 1969). In
a non-human primate model, CC sometimes led to delay in folliculogenesis
with a lengthening of ovulation intervals (Marut and Hodgen, 1982).
Despite elevated gonadotrophin levels, oestrogen levels were decreased,
suggesting ovarian refractoriness in the presence of CC. It is postulated that
CC, via its anti-oestrogenic properties, inhibits induction of gonadotrophin
receptors within the ovary, and may lead to abnormal ovulatory mechan-

isms. However, this is not entirely clear since recent in vitro work showed that CC can enhance induction of follicle-stimulating hormone (FSH) and luteinizing hormone (LH) receptors (Kessel and Hsueh, 1987). Therefore the exact mechanisms of CC action within the ovary and follicle remain to be clarified. Future work needs to address: the racemic mixtures of En and ZU isomers (see below) and their individual effects on the ovary; the role of follicular peptides, such as inhibin (McLachlan et al, 1987) and follicle regulatory protein (di Zerega et al, 1983), as induced by CC; the further characterization of the hypothalamic–pituitary site of action of CC, as related to central neurotransmitters (i.e. opiates; Judd et al, 1987), immunoreactive gonadotrophin levels and bioactive gonadotrophin levels (Tenover et al, 1987).

The endometrium is another potential target site for CC and may contribute to manifestation of luteal phase abnormalities. CC competes with oestradiol for binding to cytosol receptors (Bowman et al, 1981) and may also suppress oestradiol receptor synthesis (Kurl and Morris, 1978). When receptors were measured in human endometrium after CC therapy, oestradiol receptor concentrations were lower compared to normal controls (Aksel et al, 1986). Therefore, luteal phase defects during CC therapy may result from either ovarian or endometrial endpoints. If a luteal phase defect is uncovered by endometrial biopsy, monitoring with both hormonal indicators and sonographic determination of follicular growth is recommended. If abnormal folliculogenesis is determined, then the ovulation induction protocol should be modified; if ovulatory mechanisms appear normal, therapy with supplemental progesterone should be directed towards the endometrium.

A second area of concern with CC treatment relates to effects on the oocyte. For the past few years, CC in combination with human menopausal gonadotrophin (hMG) has been the main stimulation protocol for in vitro fertilization (IVF), used predominantly in the UK, Australia and France. However, evidence now suggests that CC may exert deleterious effects on oocytes and subsequent blastocyst formation. In the rat, degenerative changes were noted in the oocyte in culture (Laufer et al, 1982). In mice, CC led to a decreased number of ovulated oocytes, decreased embryo development, and an increase in degenerated ova (Laufer et al, 1983). Similar effects were seen in in vitro perfused rabbit ovaries (Yoshimura et al, 1986), an effect that was reversed by administration of oestradiol (Yoshimura et al, 1987). The clinical sequelae to this remain to be determined, however it is possible that fertility is impaired due to direct oocyte or embryo toxic events, regardless of whether fertilization takes place in vivo or in vitro. It may not be possible to avoid this problem during routine administration for ovulation induction. Newer agents with different formulations, different pharmacokinetics, or differing regimens for use may be necessary in the future. Many in vitro fertilization programmes have changed from CC regimens to combination protocols with gonadotrophin-releasing hormone (GnRH) agonist and hMG (see below): comparison trials between standard regimens and newer protocols will be forthcoming.

A corollary to the above concerns related to oocyte development is the question of birth defects with CC treatment. There is surely an increased incidence of spontaneous abortion in CC-treated women, although some of this may be due to earlier monitoring of pregnancy in these individuals. The incidence of congenital abnormalities gathered to date does not appear to be increased (Kurachi et al, 1983), however, recent studies have drawn attention to this concern. When human female genital tissue was implanted into mice treated with CC or tamoxifen, the second major anti-oestrogen, teratogenic effects were noted in these genital tissues. These effects were similar to those seen with administration of diethylstilboestrol (Cuhna et al, 1987). Similarly, in another study in female mice, tamoxifen again led to abnormal genital changes (Taguchi and Nishizuka, 1985). These studies, although not directly applicable to the human situation, stress the need for continued understanding of in vivo anti-oestrogen effects on the growing fetus, and the need for careful clinical follow-up of female infants born after ovulation induction with these agents. Inadvertent exposure of these drugs during pregnancy should be avoided.

Even when properly administered, it is clear that the half-life of CC is prolonged and may affect a developing fetus. In general, the half-life is approximately 5–7 days. Radioactivity, after an oral tracer dose, may be detected in the faeces from up to 6 weeks (Schreiber et al, 1966). Using a radioreceptor assay, in patients receiving CC on days 5–9 of the cycle, activity was present in some patients on day 22, but in none 60 days after treatment (Geier et al, 1987).

The pharmacokinetics of the racemic mixtures of CC have also been studied. CC contains two isomers with approximately 38% zuclomiphene (cis) and 62% enclomiphene (trans). The ZU isomer was detected up to 1 month after treatment (Mikkelson et al, 1986). The ZU form is relatively oestrogenic and enclomiphene is anti-oestrogenic, but the exact effects of these isomers remain to be determined in the future. Both isomers may adversely affect mouse oocytes fertilized in vitro and in vivo (Schmidt et al, 1986). It has been shown that when the agonistic or antagonistic oestrogenic properties of CC are evaluated, the exact endpoint must be well defined (Clark and Geuthrie, 1981). Therefore, they may be different for hypothalamic, ovarian, or endometrial effects. Once this is understood, new racemic formations may be derived and tailored to the appropriate clinical situation, perhaps even individually for patients.

This racemic differentiation also remains true in the treatment of malignancies. Anti-oestrogens, mostly tamoxifen, have been used as adjuvant therapy for breast cancer in the post-menopausal women. Tamoxifen causes an oestrogen-like decrease in gonadotrophin levels without an effect on steroid levels, but the exact mechanism of action is not known. The drug consists of a racemic mixture of isomers, but, in the treatment of breast cancer, it appears that only the trans-tamoxifen is active (Robertson et al, 1982). Recent studies have described the growth-inhibiting effect on breast cancer cells in vitro, and that trans-tamoxifen regulated RNA transcription and turnover (Benz and Santos, 1987). In the future, with cDNA probes, a greater understanding of this mechanism will be forthcoming. In addition, newer compounds continue to be developed; one triphenylethylene compound, Fc-1157a, almost a pure anti-oestrogen in the rat uterus, is undergoing clinical trials for efficacy and shows promise (Kangas et al, 1986).

Some investigators suggest that tamoxifen or related compounds should be used as an adjunct for prevention of breast cancer in certain high-risk women, since it can prevent the induction of rat mammary cancer (Jordan, 1976). However, the long-term effects are not known; concerns arise related to the administration of an anti-oestrogen in post-menopausal women when current therapy now dictates the use of oestrogen replacement therapy in most post-menopausal women for prevention of osteoporosis and for its possible cardiovascular protective effects.

Some evidence suggests that anti-oestrogens, specifically CC, may be used as a supplement to oestrogen replacement therapy. Clinically, CC successfully protected the endometrium from the proliferative effects of oestrogen (Kokko et al, 1981). Withdrawal bleeding was diminished by the addition of CC. Similar endometrial effects were noted in a monkey study, with the additional finding of the conservation of urinary calcium (Abbasi and Hodgen, 1986). Clearly future studies should be directed at the long-term use of CC in combination with oestrogens or as the sole agent for hormone replacement studies, with emphasis on symptoms, bone density studies, and lipid profiles. The ideal formulation would need to protect the bone, endometrium, and heart, in addition to decreasing the incidence of breast cancer in post-menopausal women.

## ANTIPROGESTINS

The clinical availability of progesterone antagonists is another major breakthrough in the reproductive sciences, providing potential new treatments and probes for reproductive physiology understanding. Previous chapters have outlined the current status of these agents for menstrual induction, interruption of pregnancy and obstetrical indications. Here, future areas for research and speculation on several clinical utilities are included.

The spectrum of compounds with anti-progestational activity has been limited. Mifepristone (RU486; Roussell-Uclaf), a non-steroid derivative with potent anti-progestin and anti-glucocorticoid activity, is the prototype drug for this class of compounds. However, this agent is the first generation, and with greater understanding of the pharmacology and endocrinology of this group of drugs, newer analogues are being developed which may be more specific for particular disease states. It is already known that mifepristone is not a pure antagonist, but it clearly has some progesterone agonist actions (Collins and Hodgen, 1986; Koering et al, 1986); in addition, due to the similarity between the progesterone and glucocorticoid receptors, mifepristone has both anti-progesterone and anti-glucocorticoid activity. Currently under study is a new anti-progestin, ZK 98734, a compound with substantially less affinity for the glucocorticoid receptor (Henderson, 1987). Therefore, although most of the present discussion focuses on mifepristone, it should be borne in mind that this is only the first of many anti-progestins to become available.

Certainly the most exciting, although highly controversial, potential use of mifepristone is in early-pregnancy termination. Mifepristone has demonstrated efficacy as a contragestive agent for interruption of pregnancy. Success as a once-a-month contraceptive appears more limited. As a contragestive, this medical termination of pregnancy is a major breakthrough for reproductive regulation. Success rates are as high as 92% when administered within 41 days of the last menstrual period; however, more studies have shown abortion rates up to approximately 85% when mifepristone was used alone. It has puzzled many investigators that pregnancy terminations have not approached 100% effectiveness when mifepristone was properly administered early in pregnancy. Future research needs to define optimum dose and time of administration, although increasing dose has led to increased success rates (Mishell et al, 1987). Already rates have been increased by adding uterotonic drugs, such as prostaglandin $E_2$ (Bygdeman and Swahn, 1985; see Chapter 7).

One problem with the delivery of mifepristone may be the high degree of plasma protein binding exhibited in humans; approximately 93% of mifepristone is protein-bound, presumably to $\alpha$-1 acid glycoprotein (AAG), and to a much lesser extent to albumin (Kawai et al, 1987). In vivo rat uterine uptake studies demonstrate the difficulty of extraction of the drug out of the vasculature, due to this high-affinity binding. It is also clear that there is a wide range of AAG levels in normal and pregnant patients, since AAG is an acute-phase reactant (Steingold et al, 1987c). Therefore, one could postulate that some of the failures of mifepristone as a contragestive may be due to diminished bioavailability of mifepristone to uterine target sites as a result of elevated AAG levels.

Future studies may address the effect of combination therapy with agents known to bind to AAG, to compete effectively for AAG binding sites and to increase the concentration of free mifepristone (Steingold et al, 1988). The mode of administration also requires evaluation since a significant degree of metabolism occurs with oral administration. Primate studies have demonstrated limited effectiveness of vaginal (Hodgen, 1985) and intramuscular delivery of mifepristone (Chillik et al, 1986). Further studies should also assess the role of alternative parenteral formulations to avoid the first-pass hepatic effects.

As a luteal-phase contraceptive, results have not been highly promising. Attempts have utilized mifepristone as an immediate post-coital contraceptive: to induce menstruation, the drug must be administered during the luteal phase. Studies must address efficacy as a 'morning-after' pill. A more interesting question is whether anti-progestins may be effective in a combination oral contraceptive. Commonly used progestins in the oral contraceptives cause unwanted hepatic effects, including adverse lipoprotein profiles. If anti-progestins can successfully block ovulation and implantation (with or without oestrogen therapy), future studies can then assess the effects on hepatic parameters as a potential contraceptive.

An interesting corollary that remains to be explored is the use of anti-progestins, in combination with oestrogens, as hormone replacement therapy for the post-menopausal women. Preliminary studies in both non-human primates (Koering et al, 1986) and humans (Gravanis et al, 1985) have demonstrated that mifepristone has some progestomimetic effects on oestrogen-primed endometrium. Therefore these agents may be able to prevent effectively endometrial proliferation and hyperplastic changes, due to this anti-mitogenic action on oestrogen-induced changes. Again, metabolic studies are necessary to evaluate the potential advantages of the anti-progestins compared with true progestational agents in the menopausal women.

Another similar utilization of anti-progestins may be in the treatment of endometriosis. From this known anti-mitogenic action on endometrium, preliminary studies evaluated the effects on ectopic endometrium in monkeys with endometriosis (Hodgen, unpublished data). Ovulation was inhibited in these animals and serum levels of oestradiol, progesterone and gonadotrophins were suppressed. Post-treatment evaluation revealed improvement of endometriotic implants and ovarian endometriomas among a series of monkeys with moderate to severe endometriosis. Clinical trials are in order to evaluate this potentially important clinical application of these anti-progestational agents.

One aspect not yet completely understood is the consequence of long-term administration of anti-progestins. Most of the studies to date utilize mifepristone in short courses of therapy, mainly as a contragestive. If chronic therapy is contemplated, extensive safety studies need to be done to elucidate the metabolic and biochemical effect of at least a 6-month treatment course.

There are other potential applications of long-term treatment. For example, mifepristone displays moderate affinity for the androgen receptor and has some anti-androgenic activity (Philibert et al, 1985). Chronic administration could lead to suppression of androgen levels and decreased androgenic action with possible efficacy in the treatment of hirsutism and polycystic ovary disease. Due to its anti-glucocorticoid activity, preliminary trials have already suggested successful treatment of Cushing's syndrome (Nieman et al, 1985).

Finally, the role of anti-progestins as an adjunct to labour induction needs to be clarified. Due to presumed myometrial effects, mifepristone can cause fetal expulsion in cases of intrauterine deaths (Cabrol et al, 1985). Accelerated cervical ripening has also been reported (Frydman et al, 1986). In monkey studies, mifepristone in combination with oxytocin proved effective for cervical dilation and labour induction; indeed it was more effective than mifepristone or oxytocin alone (Wolf et al, 1988b). However, concerns exist related to transplacental passage of mifepristone or its metabolites to the developing fetus. In monkey studies, rapid equilibration of mifepristone was noted between maternal and fetal compartments, suggesting simple diffusion (Wolf et al, 1988a). No acute toxicity was noticed; clearly this issue needs careful analysis with long-term neonatal follow-up, including data indicating the normality of pituitary, gonadal and adrenal function.

There are surely other indications that remain to be explored; anti-progestins may manifest progestin, anti-androgen or anti-glucocorticoid activity, depending on the precise hormonal milieu. The coming generation of anti-progestins will allow greater flexibility in matching the desired actions with the endpoints sought.

## LHRH ANALOGUES

The elucidation of the structure of LHRH, the development of analogues and the modifications of the structure of LHRH were major advances in the understanding and treatment of many reproductive endocrine diseases. The availability of highly potent agonists and antagonists of LHRH now provides the practitioner with effective tools to inhibit significantly gonadal steroid production. This section will provide a framework for specific disease states from which the reader can understand the vast potential for clinical use.

The analogues of LHRH may be either agonists or antagonists, with reference to their initial effects on gonadotrophin release. Agonists cause a transient, rapid and usually enhanced release of LH and FSH from the pituitary gland; with continued stimulation of the gonadotropes however, a pituitary desensitization occurs whereby release of gonadotrophins is inhibited (Heber et al, 1982; Keri et al, 1983; Werlin and Hodgen, 1983). The initial stimulatory phase is variable but is approximately 2 weeks. The antagonistic analogues have a high affinity for the gonadotrophin receptors, but are without biological activity (Cetel et al, 1983; Kenigsberg et al, 1984a,b; Chillik et al, 1987). Therefore, gonadotrophin suppression is manifested within 1 day. The end-result of both agonist and antagonist treatment is a marked decrease in serum gonadotrophin levels with resultant suppression of gonadal steroidogenesis. The disadvantages of the agonists are the initial stimulatory phase and the prolonged time to suppression compared with the agonist. However, agonist drugs are currently available for use, whereas clinical trials for antagonists are still in the early stages due to problems with histamine release and potential allergic reactions. Newer antagonists, currently being evaluated, show greater promise for clinical use (Chillik et al, 1987).

One of the first trials performed with a LHRH agonist was in the treatment of true precocious puberty (Crowley et al, 1981). This still remains one of the best indications for this group of compounds. In gonadotrophin-sensitive true precocious puberty, agonists can provide complete suppression of gonadal steroid production in both males and females and a cessation of secondary sexual characteristics. The major flaw with most previously available treatments has been the lack of effect on the growth spurt, and the ultimate short stature of these patients. Preliminary reports with the LHRH agonists appear to show a decrease in growth velocity, allowing chronological age to approximate bone age (Comite et al, 1986). If these interpretations remain valid, such compounds will be the drug of choice for true precocious puberty. This has also provided an understanding for the mechanisms involved in the initiation of this disease state, allowing differentiation of gonadotrophin-dependent and non-dependent processes. In contrast, it is now clear that McCune–Albright disease is not dependent on the normal activation of the hypothalamic–pituitary axis, and other mechanisms must be in operation (Foster et al, 1984).

The exact mechanism of action of the desensitization induced by LHRH analogues has not been entirely clarified. Initially believed to be a gonadotroph receptor phenomenon, the process may not correlate with receptor binding, and is substantially more complicated (Keri et al, 1983). A very recent exciting observation may shed further light on this area. The treatment of hypogonadal women with a LHRH antagonist resulted in a significant decrease in bioactive serum FSH levels, while immunoreactive FSH levels were relatively unchanged (Dahl et al, 1988). Characterization of these immunoreactive FSH moities provided evidence for the existence of FSH antagonism by certain isoforms, as demonstrated in vitro by granulosa cell assay. The implications of these findings are manifold. Firstly, a postulated mechanism of action of the LHRH antagonist relates to changing of the bioactive:immunoreactive ratio of FSH, changes possibly due to glycosylation. Secondly, this study demonstrates the occurrence of a naturally occurring circulating anti-hormone. It is possible that pathophysiological hypogonadal conditions may be aetiologically related to these circulating hormones. Finally, characterization of these anti-hormones may provide the pharmacological understanding for the development of new anti-reproductive compounds.

Endometriosis is another exciting potential use of LHRH analogues. Using a potent agonist, these patients can be reversibly suppressed to castrate levels of serum oestrogens, a hormonal milieu known to be suppressive to endometriotic implants (Meldrum et al, 1982). Subsequent clinical trials have proven that these drugs can be effective for treatment of endometriosis; this therapy is probably equal to the currently used medication, danazol (Werlin and Hodgen, 1983; Schriock et al, 1985; Steingold et al, 1987a; Hanzel et al, 1988). Major questions need to be resolved, however, in future clinical trials. Due to the menopausal state of these patients, significant side-effects due to oestrogen deprivation can occur, including severe hot flushes, vaginal atrophy, emotional disturbances, and the potential for calcium loss from bone. Of major concern is this possibility of bone loss and preliminary studies have shown conflicting results (Cann et al, 1986; Tummon et al, 1987). It appears, however, that this loss is temporary and reversible, but clearly more data are necessary.

Another unresolved issue is the exact regimen to be utilized for treatment of endometriosis. Do the patients need to be completely suppressed? In the monkey model, intermittent injections of LHRH agonist effectively suppressed endometriotic implants, despite allowing oestrogen levels to rise periodically (Werlin and Hodgen, 1983). This could be one manoeuvre to diminish the adverse effects of oestrogen lack. Others have added adjunctive therapies in an effort to minimize side-effects and improve efficacy. The addition of medroxyprogesterone acetate to LHRH agonist treatment for 6 months did diminish side-effects, but caused less improvement in disease as compared to agonist alone (Cedars et al, 1987). However, norethindrone supplementation showed promise in a preliminary study in that efficacy improved, hot flushes diminished and bone density was not altered (Surrey et al, 1988). Future studies will define the proper method of a treatment course of LHRH analogues in endometriosis.

A third area where LHRH agonists appear to be making an immediate impact is with ovulation induction, especially for IVF. Using this in combination with hMG may evolve into the primary stimulation protocol for IVF patients (Neveu et al, 1987). Clearly LHRH agonists (or antagonists) can suppress the unwanted LH surge which may occasionally be seen with controlled hyperstimulation. However, poor responders may also do better with this combined therapy (Serafini et al, 1988). This principle was first shown using a LHRH antagonist (Kenigsberg et al, 1984a,b). The initial suppression of the ovary to a baseline state followed by gonadotrophin stimulation provides better synchrony of follicular maturation and prevention of premature LH surges. In these early studies, pregnancy rates appear favourable and may exceed previously reported statistics in problem responders.

Other areas of ovulation induction need further study. Using a similar regimen in polycystic ovary disease, pregnancy rates were encouraging (Dodson et al, 1987). The suppression of ovarian androgen production via LHRH agonists may provide a more favourable follicular environment for these oocytes and lead to a greater contribution to pregnancy. Similarly, the perimenopausal patient needs to be studied. These patients, with elevated early follicular phase FSH levels, have impaired follicular development. It has been proposed that the elevated levels of FSH may down-regulate granulosa cell receptors, therefore prior suppression of gonadotrophins before ovulation induction has theoretical merit (Nimrod and Lamprecht, 1980). Developing an effective regimen for the perimenopausal patient is a key goal for fertility clinics worldwide, due to the increased numbers of women who have delayed childbearing and the known poor results in these patients.

Polycystic ovary disease is a fourth area of potential effectiveness. For hyperandrogenaemic states, analogues clearly inhibit the ovarian contribution to elevated testosterone and androstenedione levels (Chang et al, 1983). Clinically a 6-month treatment course provided sustained reduction in these levels, comparable to those seen in menopausal women and controls (Steingold et al, 1987b). The menopausal side-effects could be avoided by intermittent treatment with exogenous oestrogen therapy. The agonist can also reduce androgen levels both in ovarian hyperthecosis (Steingold et al, 1986) and in one report, a Leydig cell tumour (Kennedy et al, 1987). In the hyperthecosis patient, treatment with gonadotrophins was instituted after finishing the agonist, with successful induction of ovulation—an event which is very difficult in these patients with standard treatment.

Gonadotrophin suppression is also a helpful probe in trying to understand the initiating events in polycystic ovary disease. The adrenal, ovary and pituitary may all be evaluated separately. Studies have addressed the origin of serum progestins by ovarian suppression (Chetkowski et al, 1984), pituitary and ovarian recovery after suppression (De Ziegler et al, 1986), and the combined effects of gonadal and adrenal suppression (Cedars et al, 1988). The conclusions, supported by these studies, point to a basic ovarian defect in polycystic ovary disease rather than pituitary or adrenal dysfunction. The utility of analogues both in treatment and understanding disease will apply to many other disease entities.

The need for effective contraceptive agents is a major priority facing reproductive scientists today. Clearly LHRH analogues can suppress ovulation in women; clinical trials have demonstrated efficacy as an ovulation inhibitor (Berquyst et al, 1979). As mentioned above, the long-term use of these agents is questioned due to potential side-effects. Therefore the use of intermittent administration of a LHRH antagonist, as previously reported, may prevent the profound hypo-oestrogenic milieu (Kenigsberg and Hodgen, 1986). Otherwise, combination therapy is necessary. First, the dose needs to be adjusted to allow ovarian oestrogen production; however, due to this now chronic unopposed oestrogen, a progestin is necessary for endometrial protection (Lemay et al, 1987). This somewhat unwieldy approach shows the difficulty in balancing efficacy with safe side-effects.

There are numerous other potential indications for LHRH analogues. Hormone-dependent tumours, for example prostate cancer, are improved with agonist treatment; this avoids surgical orchidectomy (Smith et al, 1985). Agonist therapy leads to suppression of the fibroid uterus, but resumption of growth apparently occurs after cessation of treatment (Coddington et al, 1986). Therefore, the exact role of these agents has not been defined.

A LHRH antagonist has been proposed as a testing procedure to predict the predisposition to osteoporosis; clinical studies need to substantiate these tests (Abassi and Hodgen, 1986). Finally, studies need to address the potential for gamete sparing prior to chemotherapy for malignancies. It is well known that certain chemotherapeutics, specifically alkylating agents, may irreversibly destroy germ cells. It is possible that gonadal suppression to a quiescent state may afford protection.

The future of these agents depends on determining the ideal mode of administration and defining adjunctive therapies; the potential for side-effects needs to be clarified. Newer delivery forms are currently being developed. Long-acting injections, with microspheres or depot forms, can avoid the need for the daily administration of these agents. Although LHRH analogues remain one of the major advances in reproductive therapies in recent years, there is still much work to be done in defining the most appropriate applications.

## ANTI-ANDROGENS

The understanding of anti-androgenic mechanisms and actions is still relatively limited, although great strides have been made in this area of basic hormonal action. For years attempts have been made to counteract the effects of endogenous androgens for various disease states. Androgens can be suppressed by inhibiting stimulation of a steroid-producing organ (e.g. LHRH agonist) or androgen secretion can be diminished by inhibiting synthesis (e.g. aminoglutethimide). However, the most specific form of inhibition is by direct binding to the intracellular androgen receptor without overlap in binding to other steroid receptors such as a progestin, gluco-corticoid or oestrogen. With greater knowledge of receptor physiology, individual compounds can be developed with a specific affinity for the androgen receptor.

The indications for anti-androgen therapy are relatively limited. In males, the classic use is in advanced prostate cancer (Huggins and Hodges, 1941), and most of the knowledge of these agents has been derived from long-standing studies in this area. In females, syndromes of excess androgen production are frequently encountered, necessitating effective treatments. This section will focus on specific agents, rather than disease entities, and include some newer agents which may find their way into clinical use.

Cyproterone acetate (CPA), reviewed in more detail in an earlier chapter, is one of the most widely used anti-androgenic compounds worldwide, although it is not available for prescription in the USA. This compound is a potent progestational agent, but effectively inhibits androgens at the target organ (Neumann, 1977); it also has anti-gonado-trophic properties which are important for efficacy (Knuth et al, 1984). CPA has been shown to be effective for treatment in prostate cancer (Scott and Schirmer, 1966) and female hirsutism (Ismail et al, 1974). Although it appears that newer modalities may replace CPA in the adjunctive therapy in prostate cancer, CPA is still a key treatment option for hirsutism. The major question that needs to be resolved in the treatment of hirsutism is the ideal manner of administration. CPA may be given alone, either in oral or depot form, or may be given in a sequential fashion with ethinyloestradiol. In severe hirsutism, efficacy and side-effects may be similar, although the nature of the adverse effects are different (Belisle and Love, 1986). Clearly more trials are necessary to improve treatment regimens in these indi-viduals, as well as comparative studies with newer agents. Recent work has already begun on an endocrinological comparison between CPA and GnRH agonists in women with polycystic ovary disease, describing a more complete inhibition with the GnRH agonist (Couzinet et al, 1986a,b). However, clinical studies will be needed to address specifically symptomatic improvement in women—often a highly subjective endpoint.

A second major anti-androgen is the non-steroidal drug flutamide, which appears to inhibit androgen uptake or inhibit androgen receptor binding (Peets et al, 1974). The predominant use for flutamide is in the treatment of prostate cancer (Sogani et al, 1975). Although improvement in disease is noted, results have not been as encouraging as was hoped. Therefore, the current and future direction lies in the appropriate combination therapy. Flutamide is most effective when used in combination with castration, whether surgical or in combination with a LHRH agonist (Labrie et al, 1987). This combination may block progression of disease in up to one-third of patients; life expectancy is also increased.

This type of therapy also provides insight into the underlying hormonal events occurring in prostatic tissue. It was formerly believed that patients who failed castration had androgen-insensitive tumours; however, it is possible that these patients have high endogenous dihydrotestosterone levels within the prostatic tumour which prevent adequate suppression by the anti-androgenic agents. Although testicular androgens are surgically or medically removed, adrenal androgen production is still operative. Therefore, combination therapy with flutamide reduces adrenal precursors by 50%, while testicular production is completely removed (Brochu et al, 1987). These major findings will dramatically alter future treatments for prostate cancer. A tremendous benefit for the patient will be achieved if medical castration can replace surgical castration, and if combination therapy will continue to provide increased life expectancy for these patients.

A newer anti-androgenic agent which also shows a great deal of promise in the treatment of prostate cancer is anandron. This non-steroidal agent interacts with the androgen receptor and is devoid of other hormonal effects, such as anti-oestrogen or anti-progestin activity (Moguilewski et al, 1987). It contrasts with flutamide in that it requires no metabolic activitation, whereas flutamide requires conversion to the hydroxy derivative. Preliminary studies suggest that combination castration and anandron may provide symptomatic improvement and increased remissions in patients with advanced prostatic cancer, via the mechanisms discussed above (Navratil, 1987). It should be stressed that a pure anti-androgen is necessary when LHRH agonist therapy is instituted in these patients to prevent the well known flare-up response to agonists; LHRH agonists have an initial gonadal stimulation phase, with increased testosterone production, therefore receptor anti-androgens can prevent these unwanted sequelae.

An interesting but unrelated corollary to these works relates to lipoprotein profiles. When complete androgen blockade was achieved in a group of men with a LHRH agonist and anandron, serum high-density lipoprotein cholesterol increased, while low-density lipoprotein cholesterol was unchanged, leading to a favourable atherogenic ratio (Moorjani et al, 1987). These endocrinological perturbations will allow future studies to ascertain the relative risks of androgens and oestrogens in the development of cardiovascular disease, and possibly appropriate hormonal manipulation will be able to decrease those risks effectively.

In the USA, excess androgen production in women is frequently treated with spironolactone (Biosselle and Tremblay, 1979); this therapy is probably second only to oral contraceptive suppression for treatment of hirsutism in this country. However, the mechanism of action of spironolactone still requires further definition. It may increase the metabolic clearance of testosterone and increase conversion of testosterone to oestradiol (Rose et al, 1977). Testosterone synthesis may be diminished, presumably by inhibition of 17-hydroxylase and 17-20-lyase activity (Givens, 1985). Furthermore, spironolactone may provide direct receptor antagonism and interfere with translocation of the dihydrotestosterone receptor complex into the nucleus (Rittmaster and Loriaux, 1987). The effects on adrenal steroidogenesis are variable, but adrenal androgen production is probably not dramatically altered (Serafini and Lobo, 1985). Therefore, spironolactone has a multifaceted mechanism of action. Its net effect is an overall suppression of androgen activity with impressive clinical results to date.

Studying the effects of spironolactone has provided further understanding of peripheral tissue events in the aetiology of hirsutism. Current theory suggests that serum 3α-diol glucuronide (3α-diol G) is a reliable marker for hirsutism in many individuals (Lobo et al, 1983). However, with spironolactone treatment, the 3α-diol G pathway may be a disposal mechanism for testosterone and dihydrotestosterone metabolism, and measurement of this hormone may not be a reliable marker while the patient is on spironolactone treatment (Lobo et al, 1985). Clearly, understanding these peripheral tissue events will allow for better understanding of the pathogenesis of clinical states in which exaggerated responses to circulating (or peripheral) hormone levels are noted. Further experimentation will aim at developing compounds which may directly inhibit events at the receptor level and subsequent metabolism.

There are also numerous agents that may inhibit androgen biosynthesis at various sites along the steroidogenic pathway. One agent increasingly being studied is the orally active anti-fungal agent, ketoconazole (Sonino, 1987). It was initially observed that men taking this medication developed gynaecomastia and subsequent work showed a decrease in serum testosterone levels (Pont et al, 1982). Ketoconazole inhibits certain cytochrome P450-mediated systems in both testicular and ovarian tissue, with reduction in 17 hydroxylase, 17-20 lyase, 3β hydroxysteroid dehydrogenase, and possibly aromatase activity (Di Mattina et al, 1988). The overall result is a reduction in serum androgen levels, and studies are now beginning to address the role of ketoconazole as treatment as an anti-androgen. Preliminary studies have provided encouragement for the study of prostate cancer (Denis et al, 1985), precocious puberty (Holland et al, 1985) and hirsutism (Carvalho et al, 1985). In addition, ketoconazole has been used as a potential treatment of Cushing's disease (Sonino et al, 1985). However, due to the potency of this agent, careful study needs to be conducted to evaluate adverse effects during a long-term treatment course. Drugs of this nature are certainly in their infancy, and more studies are forthcoming.

Finally, newer agents are being evaluated which affect other sites of action. The enzyme, 5α reductase, converts testosterone to dihydrotestosterone. As alluded to above, dihydrotestosterone is important for the cellular events associated with androgen action. Clearly, inhibition of 5α reductase activity would be an important and effective modality for inhibition of androgen effects. Epitestosterone is the 17α-hydroxy epimer of testosterone, a natural metabolite, and causes 5α reductase inhibition (Nuck and Lucky, 1987). Animal studies show that epitestosterone is an effective anti-androgen and further studies may evaluate potential clinical safety and effectiveness. Other 5α reductase inhibitors remain to be studied (Vacquez et al, 1987).

Thus, clinically effective anti-androgenic agents are needed to treat pathological states both in males and females. As always, understanding of the basic physiology relating to hormone synthesis, uptake, receptor binding, and cellular metabolism is critical to the development of pharmacological intervention. Newer compounds are being developed that can interact at any number of the sites of androgen action. Both safety and availability of chronic administration are prerequisites for the utilization of these compounds. Finally, with greater understanding of the molecular events of androgen action, a molecular basis for therapy can be envisaged. Nucleic acid (cDNA) probes may be developed that can prevent androgen processing and secretion, leading to newer, more specific anti-androgen modalities.

## OXYTOCIN ANTAGONISTS

A final reproductive anti-hormone category which may have important future implications is oxytocin antagonism. Prematurity remains a major cause of neonatal morbidity and mortality, and effective treatment of premature labour is of paramount importance. Recent work has addressed the issue of oxytocin antagonist, from developmental stage to initial clinical trial. A promising competitive antagonist of oxytocin is a vasotocin derivative 1-deamino-[D-Tyr (Oethyl)$^2$, Thr$^4$, Orn$^8$] vasotocin (ORF 22164). In vitro and in vivo animal studies have reported an effective decrease in uterine contractility (Hahn et al, 1987). An initial pilot study in 13 women described promising results with this agent for inhibition of premature uterine contractions (Akerlund et al, 1987). Clearly, future studies with oxytocin antagonists will allow further understanding of the pathogenesis of certain types of premature labour as well as the possibility for effective therapy.

## SUMMARY

Anti-hormones are important in reproductive medicine because they are useful tools that teach us about the normal physiological actions of hormones. They also provide effective therapies to control or treat a variety of pathogenic processes. We expect that the future repertoire of anti-hormones will include the paracrine and autocrine regulators of specific cell functions, in addition to the endocrine systems described here. The availability of recombinant DNA expression systems for an ever larger portion of the human genome will surely accelerate the development of novel anti-hormones.

## REFERENCES

Abbasi R & Hodgen GD (1986) Predicating the predisposition to osteoporosis: gonadotropin-releasing hormone antagonist for acute estrogen deficiency test. *Journal of the American Medical Association* **255**: 1600.

Akerlund M, Stromberg P, Hauksson A et al (1987) Inhibition of uterine contractions of premature labour with an oxytocin analogue. Results from a pilot study. *British Journal of Obstetrics and Gynaecology* **94**: 1040.

Aksel S, Saracoglu OF, Weoman RR & Weibe RH (1986) Effects of clomiphene citrate on cytosolic estradiol and progesterone receptors concentrations in secretory endometrium. *American Journal of Obstetrics and Gynecology* **155:** 1219.

Belisle S & Love EJ (1986) Clinical efficacy and safety of cyproterone acetate in severe hirsutism. Results of a multicentered Canadian study. *Fertility and Sterility* **46:** 1015.

Benz C & Santos GF (1987) Effects of cis and trans tamoxifen isomers on RNA incorporation of human breast cancer cells. *Molecular Pharmacology* **32:** 13.

Berquyst C, Millius SJ & Wide L (1979) Inhibition of ovulation in women by intranasal treatment with a luteinizing hormone releasing hormone agonist. *Contraception* **19:** 497.

Biosselle A & Tremblay RR (1979) New therapeutic approach to the hirsute patient. *Fertility and Sterility* **32:** 276.

Bowman SP, Leake A & Morris ID (1981) Time-related effects of enclomiphene upon central and peripheral oestrogen target tissues and cytoplasmic receptors. *Journal of Endocrinology* **89:** 117.

Brochu M, Belanger A, Dupont A, Cusan L & Labrie F (1987) Effects of flutamide and aminoglutethimide on plasma 5-α-reduced steroid glucuronide concentrations in castrated patients with cancer of the prostate. *Journal of Steroid Biochemistry* **28:** 619.

Bygdeman M & Swahn M-L (1985) Progesterone receptor blockage: effect on uterine contractibility and early pregnancy. *Contraception* **32:** 45.

Cabrol D, Bouvier, T'Yvoire M et al (1985) Induction of labour with mifepristone after intrauterine fetal death [letter]. *Lancet* **ii:** 1019.

Cann CR, Henzl M, Burry K et al (1986) Reversible bone losses induced by GnRH agonist. Abstract 24, *Endocrine Society*, June, 1986.

Carvalho D, Pignatelli D & Resende C (1985) Ketoconazole for hirsutism. *Lancet* **ii:** 560.

Cedars M, Steingold K, Lu J et al (1987) Treatment of endometriosis with a long-acting GnRH agonist and medroxyprogesterone acetate. Abstract 289, *Society for Gynecologic Investigation*, March, 1987.

Cedars M, De Ziegler D, Steingold K et al (1988) Assessment of the role of abnormal adrenal androgen metabolism and the development of ovarian dysfunction present in polycystic ovarian disease. Abstract 388, *Society for Gynecologic Investigation*, March, 1988.

Cetel MS, Rivier J, Vale W & Wen SSC (1983) The dynamics of gonadotropin inhibition in women induced by an antagonistic analog of gonadotropin-releasing hormone. *Journal of Clinical Endocrinology and Metabolism* **57:** 62.

Chang RJ, Laufer LR, Meldrum DR et al (1983) Steroid secretion in polycystic ovarian disease after ovarian suppression by a long acting gonadotropin-releasing hormone agonist. *Journal of Clinical Endocrinology and Metabolism* **56:** 897.

Chetkowski RJ, Chang RJ, Defazio J, Meldrum DR & Judd HL (1984) Origin of serum progestins and polycystic ovarian disease. *Obstetrics and Gynecology* **64:** 27.

Chillik CF, Hsiu JG, Acosta AA, van Uem JFHM & Hodgen GD (1986) RU 486 induced menses in cynomolgus monkeys: uniformity of endometrial sluffing. *Fertility and Sterility* **45:** 708.

Chillik CF, Itskovitz J, Hahn DW et al (1987) Characterizing pituitary response to a gonadotropin-releasing hormone antagonist in monkeys: tonic follicle stimulating hormones/luteinizing hormone secretion versus acute GnRH challenge tests before, during and after treatment. *Fertility and Sterility* **48:** 480.

Clark JH & Geuthrie SC (1981) Agonistic and antagonistic effects of clomiphene and its isomers. *Biology of Reproduction* **25:** 667.

Coddington CC, Collins RN, Shawker TH et al (1986) A long-acting gonadotropin-releasing hormone analog used to treat uteri. *Fertility and Sterility* **45:** 624.

Collins RL & Hodgen GD (1986) Blockade of the spontaneous midcycle gonadotropin surge in monkeys by RU 486: a progesterone antagonist or agonist? *Journal of Clinical Endocrinology and Metabolism* **63:** 1270.

Comite F, Cassorla F, Barnes KM et al (1986) Luteinizing hormone releasing hormone analog therapy for central precocious puberty. *Journal of the American Medical Association* **255:** 2613.

Couzinet P, Le Start N, Brailly S & Schaison G (1986a) Comparative effects of cyproterone acetate or a long acting gonadotropin-releasing hormone agonist in polycystic ovarian disease. *Journal of Clinical Endocrinology and Metabolism* **63:** 1031.

Couzinet P, Le Start N, Ulmann A, Baulieu EE & Schaison G (1986b) Termination of early pregnancy by the progesterone antagonist RU 486 (mifepristone). *New England Journal of Medicine* **315:** 1565.

Crowley WF, Comite F, Vale W et al (1981) Therapeutic use of pituitary desensitization with a long-acting LH-RH agonist: a potential new treatment of idiopathic precocious puberty. *Journal of Clinical Endocrinology and Metabolism* **52:** 370.

Cuhna GR, Taguchi O, Namikawa R, Nishizuka Y & Robboy SJ (1987) Teratogenic effects of clomiphene, tamoxifen and diethylstilbestrol on the developing human female genital tract. *Human Pathology* **18:** 1132.

Dahl KD, Bicsak TA & Hsueh AJW (1988) Naturally occurring antihormones: secretion of FSH antagonists by women treated with a GnRH analog. *Science* **239:** 72.

Denis L, Chaban M & Mahler C (1985) Clinical applications of ketoconazole in prostatic cancer. *Progress in Clinical and Biologic Research* **185A:** 319.

De Ziegler D, Steingold K, Cedars M et al (1986) Hormone secretion patterns in polycystic ovarian disease during recovery from chronic ovarian suppression by a GnRH agonist. Abstract 28, *American Fertility Society*, September, 1986.

Di Mattina M, Maronian N, Ashby H, Loriaux DL & Albertson BD (1988) Ketoconazole inhibit multiple steroidogenic enzymes involved in androgen biosynthesis in the human ovary. *Fertility and Sterility* **49:** 62.

di Zerega GS, Campeau JD, Nakamura RM et al (1983) Activity of a human follicular fluid protein(s) during normal and stimulated ovarian cycles. *Journal of Clinical Endocrinology and Metabolism* **57:** 838.

Dodson WC, Hughes CL, Whitesides DM et al (1987) The effect of leuprolide acetate on ovulation induction with human menopausal gonadotropin in polycystic ovary syndrome. *Journal of Clinical Endocrinology and Metabolism* **65:** 95.

Foster CM, Comite F, Pescovitz OH et al (1984) Variable response to a long-acting agonist of luteinizing hormone releasing hormone in girls with McCune–Albright Syndrome. *Journal of Clinical Endocrinology and Metabolism* **59:** 801.

Frydman R, Taylor S, Fernandez H et al (1986) Obstetrical indication of mifepristone (RU 486). *Society for Advances in Contraception*, September, 1986.

Garcia J, Jones GS & Wentz AC (1977) The use of clomiphene citrate. *Fertility and Sterility* **28:** 707.

Geier A, Lunenfeld B, Pariente C et al (1987) Estrogen receptor binding material in blood of patients after clomiphene citrate administration: determination by a radio-receptor assay. *Fertility and Sterility* **46:** 778.

Givens JR (1985) Treatment of hirsutism with spironolactone. *Fertility and Sterility* **43:** 841.

Gravanis A, Schaison G, George M et al (1985) Endometrial and pituitary responses to the steroidal antiprogestin RU 486 in post-menopausal women. *Journal of Clinical Endocrinology and Metabolism* **60:** 156.

Hahn DW, Demarist KT, Ericson E et al (1987) Evaluation of 1-deamin-[D-Tyr (Oethyl),$^2$Thr$^4$, Orn$^8$] vasotocin, an oxytocin antagonist, in animal models of uterine contractility and preterm labor: a new tocolytic agent. *American Journal of Obstetrics and Gynecology* **157:** 977.

Hanzel MR, Corson SL, Moghissi K et al (1988) Administration of nasal nafarelin as compared with oral danazol for endometriosis: a multi-centered double-line comparative clinical trial. *New England Journal of Medicine* **318:** 45.

Heber D, Dodson R, Stoskopf C, Peterson M & Swerdloff RS (1982) Pituitary desensitization and the regulation of pituitary gonadotropin-releasing hormone receptors following chronic administration of a super active GnRH analog in testosterone. *Life Sciences* **30:** 2301.

Henderson D (1987) Antiprogestational and antiglucocorticoid activities of some novel 11b-aryl substituted steroids. In Furr BJA & Wakeling AE (eds) *Pharmacology and Clinical Uses of Inhibitors of Hormone Secretion and Action*, pp 184–211. London: Baillière Tindall.

Hodgen GD (1985) Pregnancy prevention by intravaginal delivery of progesterone antagonist: RU 486 tampon for menstrual induction and absorption. *Fertility and Sterility* **454:** 263.

Holland FJ, Fishman L, Bailey JD & Fazekas ATA (1985) Ketoconazole in the management of precocious puberty not responsive to LHRH analog therapy. *New England Journal of Medicine* **312:** 1023.

Huggins C & Hodges CV (1941) Studies of prostate cancer. I. Effect of castration, estrogen and androgen injections on serum phosphatases in metastatic carcinoma of the prostate. *Cancer Research* **1**: 293.

Ismail AA, Davidson DW, Souka AR et al (1974) The evaluation of the role of androgens and hirsutism and the use of a new antiandrogen cyproterone acetate for therapy. *Journal of Clinical Endocrinology and Metabolism* **39**: 81.

Jordan VC (1976) Effect of tamoxifen on initiation and growth of DMBA-induced rate mammary carcinomata. *European Journal of Cancer* **12**: 419.

Judd SJ, Alderman J, Bowden J & Michailov L (1987) Evidence against the involvement of opiate neurons in mediating the effect of clomiphene of gonadotropin-releasing hormone neurons. *Fertility and Sterility* **47**: 574.

Kangas L, Nieminen AL, Blamco G et al (1986) A new triphenylethylene compound, FC-1157a. *Cancer Chemotherapy and Pharmacology* **17**: 109.

Kawai S, Nieman LK, Brandon DD et al (1987) Pharmacokinetic properties of the anti-glucocorticoid and antiprogesterone steroid RU 486 in man. *Journal of Pharmacology and Experimental Therapeutics* **241**: 401.

Kenigsberg D & Hodgen GD (1986) Ovulation inhibition by administration of weekly gonadotropin-releasing hormone antagonist. *Journal of Clinical Endocrinology and Metabolism* **62**: 734.

Kenigsberg D, Littman BA & Hodgen GD (1984a) Medical hypophysectomy: I. Dose–response using a gonadotropin-releasing hormone antagonist. *Fertility and Sterility* **42**: 112.

Kenigsberg D, Littman BA, Williams RF & Hodgen GD (1984b) Medical hypophysectomy: II. Variability of ovarian response to gonadotropin therapy. *Fertility and Sterility* **42**: 116.

Kennedy L, Traub AI, Atkinson AB & Sheridan B (1987) Short-term administration of gonadotropin-releasing hormone analog to a patient with a testosterone secreting ovarian. *Journal of Clinical Endocrinology and Metabolism* **64**: 1320.

Keri G, Nikolics K, Teplan I & Molnar J (1983) Desensitization of luteinizing hormone release in cultured pituitary cells by gonadotropin-releasing hormone. *Molecular and Cellular Endocrinology* **30**: 109.

Kessel B & Hsueh AJW (1987) Clomiphene citrate augments follicle stimulating hormone induced luteinizing hormone receptor content in cultured rat granulosa cells. *Fertility and Sterility* **47**: 334.

Knuth UA, Hano R & Nieschlag E (1984) Effect of flutamide or cyproterone acetate on pituitary and testicular hormones in normal men. *Journal of Clinical Endocrinology and Metabolism* **59**: 963.

Koering MJ, Healy DL & Hodgen GD (1986) Morphologic response of endometrium to a progesterone receptor antagonist, RU 486, in monkeys. *Fertility and Sterility* **45**: 280.

Kokko E, Janne O, Kauppila A & Vihko R (1981) Cyclic clomiphene citrate treatment lowers cytosol estrogen and progestin receptor concentrations in the endometrium of postmeno-pausal women on estrogen replacement therapy. *Journal of Clinical Endocrinology and Metabolism* **52**: 345.

Kurachi K, Aono T, Minagawa J & Miyake A (1983) Congenital malformations of newborn infants after clomiphene-induced ovulation. *Fertility and Sterility* **40**: 187.

Kurl RN & Morris ID (1978) Differential depletion of cytoplasmic high infinity oestrogen receptors after the in vivo administration of the anti-oestrogens, clomiphene, MER-25 and tamoxifen. *British Journal of Pharmacology* **62**: 487.

Labrie F, Dupont A, Giguere M et al (1987) Combination therapy with flutamide and castration (orchiectomy or LHRH agonist): the minimal endocrine therapy in both untreated and previously treated patients. *Journal of Steroid Biochemistry* **27**: 525.

Laufer N, Reich A, Braw R, Schenker JH & Tsafriri A (1982) The effect of clomiphene citrate on preovulatory rat follicles and culture. *Biology of Reproduction* **27**: 463.

Laufer N, Pratt BM, DeCherney AH et al (1983) The in vivo and in vitro effects of clomiphene citrate on ovulation, fertilization, and development of culture mouse oocytes. *American Journal of Obstetrics and Gynecology* **147**: 633.

Lemay A, Jean C & Faure N (1987) Endometrial histology during intermittent intranasal luteinizing hormone releasing hormone agonist sequentially combined with an oral progestogen as an antiovulatory contraception approach. *Fertility and Sterility* **48**: 775.

Lobo RA, Gysler M, March CM, Gobelsmann U, Mishell Jr et al (1982) Clinical and laboratory predictors response. *Fertility and Sterility* **37**: 168.

Lobo RA, Goebelsmann U & Horton R (1983) Evidence for the importance of peripheral tissue events in the development of hirsutism in polycystic ovary syndrome. *Journal of Clinical Endocrinology and Metabolism* **57**: 393.

Lobo RA, Shoupe D, Serafini P, Brinton D & Horton R (1985) The effects of two doses of spironolactone on serum androgens and anagen hair in hirsute women. *Fertility and Sterility* **43**: 200.

Marut EL & Hodgen GD (1982) Antiestrogenic action of high dose clomiphene in primates: pituitary augmentation but with ovarian attenuation. *Fertility and Sterility* **38**: 100.

McLachlan RI, Healy DL, Robertson DM, Burger HG & de Kretser DM (1987) Circulating immunoactive inhibin in the luteal phase and early gestation of woman undergoing ovulation induction. *Fertility and Sterility* **48**: 1001.

Meldrum DR, Chang RJ, Lu J et al (1982) 'Medical oophorectomy': using a long-acting GnRH agonist: a possible new approach to the treatment of endometriosis. *Journal of Clinical Endocrinology and Metabolism* **54**: 1081.

Mikkelson TJ, Kroboth PD, Cameron WJ et al (1986) Single dose pharmacokinetics of clomiphene citrate in normal volunteers. *Fertility and Sterility* **46**: 392.

Mishell DR, Shoupe D, Brenner PF et al (1987) Termination of early gestation with the antiprogestin steroid RU 486: medium versus low-dose. *Contraception* **35**: 307.

Moguilewsky M, Bertagna C & Hucher M (1987) Pharmacologic and clinical studies of the antiandrogen anandron. *Journal of Steroid Biochemistry* **27**: 871.

Moorjani S, Dupont A, Labrie F et al (1987) Increase in plasma high-density lipoprotein concentration following complete androgen blockade in men with prostatic carcinoma. *Metabolism* **36**: 244.

Navratil H (1987) Double-blind study of anandron versus placebo in stage D2 prostate cancer patients receiving buserelin. In Murphy G & Khoury S (eds) *Proceedings of the 2nd International Symposium on Cancer of the Prostate*. New York: Alan R Liss.

Neumann F (1977) Pharmacology and potential use of cyproterone acetate. *Hormone and Metabolic Research* **9**: 1.

Neveu S, Hedon B, Bringer J et al (1987) Ovarian stimulation by a combination of a gonadotropin-releasing agonist and gonadotropins for in vitro fertilization. *Fertility and Sterility* **47**: 639.

Nieman LK, Shrousos GP, Kellner C et al (1985) Successful treatment of Cushing's syndrome with the glucocorticoid antagonist RU 486. *Journal of Clinical Endocrinology and Metabolism* **61**: 536.

Nimrod A & Lamprecht SA (1980) Hormone-induced desensitization of cultured rat granulosa cells to FSH. *Biochemical and Biophysical Research Communications* **92**: 905.

Nuck BA & Lucky AW (1987) Epitestosterone: a potential new antiandrogen. *Journal of Investigative Dermatology* **89**: 209.

Peets EA, Henson MF & Neri RO (1974) On the mechanism of the antiandrogenic action of flutamide in the rat. *Endocrinology* **94**: 532.

Philibert D, Moguilesky M, Mary I et al (1985) Pharmacological profile of RU 486 in animals. In Baulieu EE & Segal SJ (eds) *The Antiprogestin Steroid RU 486 and Human Fertility Control*, pp 49–68. New York: Plenum Press.

Pont A, Williams PL, Azhar S et al (1982) Ketoconazole blocks testosterone synthesis. *Archives of Internal Medicine* **142**: 2137.

Rabau E, Serr D, Mashiach S et al (1967) Current concepts in the treatment of anovulation. *British Medical Journal* **4**: 446.

Rittmaster RS & Loriaux DL (1987) Hirsutism. *Annals of Internal Medicine* **106**: 95.

Robertson DW, Katzenellenbogen JA, Long DJ et al (1982) Tamoxifen antiestrogens—a comparison of the activity pharmacokinetics and metabolic activation of the cis and trans isomers of tamoxifen. *Journal of Steroid Biochemistry* **16**: 1.

Rose LI, Underwood RH, Newmark SR, Kisch ES & Williams GS (1977) Pathophysiology of spironolactone-induced gynecomastia. *Annals of Internal Medicine* **87**: 398.

Sammerstein J (1969) Mode of action of clomiphene. I. Inhibitory effect of clomiphene citrate on the formation of progesterone from acetate—1 $^{14}$C by human corpus luteum slices in vitro. *Acta Endocrinologica* **60**: 635.

Schmidt GH, Kim MH, Mansour R et al (1986) The effects of enclomiphene and zuclomiphene citrates on mouse embryos fertilized in vitro and in vivo. *American Journal of Obstetrics and Gynecology* **154**: 727.

Schreiber E, Johnson JE, Plotz EJ & Weiner M (1966) Studies with $^{14}$C labeled clomiphene citrate. *Clinical Research* **14:** 287.

Schriock E, Monroe SE, Henzl M, Jeffe RB (1985) Treatment of endometriosis with a potent agonist of gonadotropin-releasing hormone (nafarelin). *Fertility and Sterility* **44:** 583.

Scott WW & Schirmer HKA (1966) A new oral progestational steroid effective in treating prostatic cancer. *Transaction of the American Association of Genito-Urinary Surgeons* **58:** 54.

Serafini P & Lobo RA (1985) The effects of spironolactone on adrenal steroidogenesis in hirsute women. *Fertility and Sterility* **44:** 595.

Serafini P, Stone B, Kerin J et al (1988) An alternate approach to controlled hyperstimulation in 'poor responders': pre-treatment with a gonadotropin-releasing analog. *Fertility and Sterility* **49:** 90.

Smith JA, Glode LM, Wettlauffer JN et al (1985) Clinical effects of gonadotropin-releasing hormone analog in metastic carcinoma of the prostate. *Urology* **25:** 106.

Sogani PC, Ray B & Whitemore WF Jr (1975) Advanced prostatic carcinoma: flutamide therapy after conventional endocrine treatment. *Urology* **6:** 164.

Sonino N (1987) The use of ketoconazole as an inhibitor of steroid production. *New England Journal of Medicine* **317:** 812.

Sonino N, Boscaro N, Merola G & Mantero F (1985) Prolonged treatment of Cushing's disease by ketoconazole. *Journal of Clinical Endocrinology and Metabolism* **61:** 718.

Steingold KA, Judd HL, Nieberg RK, Lu JKH & Chang RJ (1986) Treatment of severe androgen excess due to ovarian hyperthecosis with a long-acting gonadotropin-releasing agonist. *American Journal of Obstetrics and Gynecology* **154:** 1241.

Steingold KA, Cedars M, Lu JKH et al (1987a) Treatment of endometriosis with a long-acting gonadotropin-releasing hormone agonist. *Obstetrics and Gynecology* **69:** 403.

Steingold KA, De Ziegler D, Cedars M et al (1987b) Clinical and hormonal effects of chronic gonadotropin-releasing agonist treatment in polycystic ovarian disease. *Journal of Clinical Endocrinology and Metabolism* **65:** 773.

Steingold KA, Matt DW & Hodgen GD (1987c) Effect of human pregnancy serum on the comparative bioavailability of progesterone and an antiprogesterone, RU 486, in the rat uterus versus liver. *American Fertility Society*, abstract 181, September, 1987.

Steingold KA, Rudy A, Matt DW, Hodgen GD (1988) Increasing the bioavailability of a progesterone antagonist: binding of RU 486 to α-1 acid glycoprotein and displacement by promethazine. *Society of Gynecologic Investigation*, abstract 28, March, 1987.

Surrey E, Steingold K, Cedars M et al (1988) Effects of combined norethindrone and GnRH agonist in treatment of endometriosis. *Society for Gynecologic Investigation*, abstract 452, March, 1988.

Taguchi O & Nishizuka Y (1985) Reproductive tract abnormalities in female mice treated neonatally with tamoxifen. *American Journal of Obstetrics and Gynecology* **151:** 675.

Tenover JS, Dahl KD, Hsueh AJW et al (1987) Serum bioactive and immunoreactive follicle-stimulating hormone levels and the response to clomiphene in healthy young and elderly men. *Journal of Clinical Endocrinology and Metabolism* **64:** 1103.

Tummon I, Pepping P, Rawlins R, Ali A & Dmowski P (1987) Effect of ovarian suppression with GnRH agonist or danazol on bone mineral density in endometriosis. *American Fertility Society*, abstract 3, September, 1987.

Vacquez MH, Tezon JG & Blaquier JA (1987) Studies on the mechanism of the antiandrogenic effect of a putative 5-α reductase inhibitor. *Journal of Steroid Biochemistry* **28:** 227.

Werlin LV & Hodgen GD (1983) Gonadotropin-releasing hormone agonist suppresses ovulation, menses, and endometriosis in monkeys: an individualized, intermittent regimen. *Journal of Clinical Endocrinology and Metabolism* **56:** 844.

Wolf JP, Chillik CF, Itskovitz J et al (1988a) Transplacental passage of a progesterone antagonist in monkeys. *American Journal of Obstetrics and Gynecology* (in press).

Wolf JP, Sinosich M, Ulmann A, Baulieu E, Hodgen GD (1988b) Progesterone antagonist (RU 486) for cervical dilation, labor induction and delivery in monkeys: effectiveness in combination with oxytocin. *Society for Gynecologic Investigation*, abstract 434, March, 1988.

Yoshimura Y, Hosoi Y, Atlas SJ & Wallach EE (1986) Effect of clomiphene citrate on in vitro ovulated ova. *Fertility and Sterility* **45:** 800.

Yoshimura Y, Hosoi Y, Atlas SJ et al (1987) Estradiol reserves the limiting effects of clomiphene citrate on early embryonic development in the in vitro perfused rabbit ovary. *Fertility and Sterility* **48:** 1030.

# Index

Note: Page numbers of article titles are in **bold** type.

731